POCKET PROTOCOLS FOR
Sonography Scanning

FOURTH EDITION

Adapted from:
Sonography Scanning: Principles and Protocols,
FOURTH EDITION

BETTY BATES TEMPKIN, BA, RT(R), RDMS
Ultrasound Consultant
Formerly Clinical Director of the Diagnostic Medical Sonography Program
Hillsborough Community College, Tampa, Florida

ELSEVIER
SAUNDERS

ELSEVIER
SAUNDERS

3251 Riverport Lane
St. Louis, Missouri 63043

Pocket Protocols for Sonography Scanning, Fourth Edition

ISBN: 978-1-4557-7322-0

Copyright © 2015, 2009, 1999, 1993 by Saunders, an imprint of Elsevier Inc.

Notice

Knowledge and best practice in this field are constantly changing. As new research and experience broaden our understanding, changes in research methods, professional practices, or medical treatment may become necessary.

Practitioners and researchers must always rely on their own experience and knowledge in evaluating and using any information, methods, compounds, or experiments described herein. In using such information or methods they should be mindful of their own safety and the safety of others, including parties for whom they have a professional responsibility.

With respect to any drug or pharmaceutical products identified, readers are advised to check the most current information provided (i) on procedures featured or (ii) by the manufacturer of each product to be administered, to verify the recommended dose or formula, the method and duration of administration, and contraindications. It is the responsibility of practitioners, relying on their own experience and knowledge of their patients, to make diagnoses, to determine dosages and the best treatment for each individual patient, and to take all appropriate safety precautions.

To the fullest extent of the law, neither the Publisher nor the authors, contributors, or editors, assume any liability for any injury and/or damage to persons or property as a matter of products liability, negligence or otherwise, or from any use or operation of any methods, products, instructions, or ideas contained in the material herein.

The Publisher

Executive Content Strategist: Sonya Seigafuse
Content Development Specialist: Laurie Gower
Content Coordinator: John Tomedi
Marketing Manager: Jamie Augustine
Publishing Services Manager: Jeff Patterson
Project Manager: Mary G. Stueck
Text Designer: Renée Duenow

Printed in India

Last digit is the print number: 9 8 7 6 5

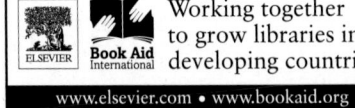

Working together
to grow libraries in
developing countries

www.elsevier.com • www.bookaid.org

POCKET PROTOCOLS FOR
Sonography Scanning

Acknowledgments

Peggy Ann Malzi Bizjak, MBA, RDMS, RT(R)(M), CRA
Radiology Manager–Ultrasound
Radiology and Medical Imaging Department
University of Virginia Health System;
Adjunct Faculty
Diagnostic Medical Sonography Program
Piedmont Virginia Community College
Charlottesville, Virginia

Amy T. Dela Cruz, MS, RDMS, RVT
Medical Sonography Program Director
South Piedmont Community College
Monroe, North Carolina

Wayne C. Leonhardt, BA, RT(R), RVT, RDMS
Faculty
Foothill College of Ultrasound
Los Altos, California;
Staff Sonographer, Technical Director, and
    Continuing Education Director
Summit Medical Center
Oakland, California

Maureen E. McDonald, BS, RDMS, RDCS
Staff Echocardiographer
Adult Echocardiography Instructor and Lecturer
Thomas Jefferson University Hospital
Philadelphia, Pennsylvania

Marsha M. Neumyer, BS, RVT, FSVU, FAIUM, ASDMS
International Director
Vascular Diagnostic Educational Services
Vascular Resource Associates
Harrisburg, Pennsylvania

Contents

PART **I**   **Introduction: Purpose and Use,** 1

PART **II**   **Image Protocol for Abnormal Sonographic Findings,** 3

PART **III** **The Abdomen,** 8

SECTION ONE ■ Image Protocols for Full Sonographic Studies of the Abdomen, 8

Liver Study With Full Abdomen, 11
Aorta Study With Full Abdomen, 33
Inferior Vena Cava Study With Full Abdomen, 59
Gallbladder and Biliary Tract Study With Full Abdomen, 82
Pancreas Study With Full Abdomen, 107

Renal Study With Full Abdomen, 131
Spleen Study With Full Abdomen, 162

SECTION TWO ■ Image Protocols for Limited Sonographic Studies of the Abdomen, 186

Aorta Study With Limited Abdomen, 188
Inferior Vena Cava Study With Limited Abdomen, 196
Right Upper Quadrant Study With Limited Abdomen, 200
Gallbladder and Biliary Tract Study With Limited Abdomen, 220
Pancreas Study With Limited Abdomen, 237
Renal Study With Limited Abdomen, 253
Spleen Study With Limited Abdomen, 267

PART IV **The Pelvis,** 273

SECTION ONE ■ Image Protocol for the Transabdominal Sonographic Study of the Female Pelvis, 273

Transabdominal Female Pelvis Study, 275

SECTION TWO ■ Image Protocol for the Transvaginal Sonographic Study of the Female Pelvis, 291

Transvaginal Female Pelvis Study, 293

SECTION THREE ■ Image Protocols for Sonographic Studies of the Male Pelvis, 307

Transrectal Prostate Gland Study, 309
Scrotum Study, 315
Penis Study, 340

PART V **Obstetrics,** 344

SECTION ONE ■ Image Protocol for the Sonographic Study of the Early First Trimester, 344

Early First Trimester Study, 346

SECTION TWO ■ Image Protocol for the Sonographic Study of the Late First Trimester, 352

Late First Trimester Study, 354

SECTION THREE ■ Image Protocol for the Sonographic Study of the Second and Third Trimesters, 359

Second and Third Trimesters Study, 361

SECTION FOUR ■ Image Protocol for the Sonographic Study of Multiple Gestations, 392

Multiple Gestations Study, 394
The Biophysical Profile, 397

PART VI **Small Parts,** 405

SECTION ONE ■ Image Protocol for the Sonographic Study of the Musculoskeletal System, 405

Musculoskeletal Study (Rotator Cuff, Carpal Tunnel, and Achilles Tendon), 407

SECTION TWO ▪ Image Protocol for the Sonographic Study of the Thyroid Gland, 419

    Thyroid Gland Study, 421

SECTION THREE ▪ Image Protocols for the Sonographic Study of the Breast, 427

    Breast Lesion Characterization, 430
    Whole Breast Study, 433

SECTION FOUR ▪ Image Protocol for the Sonographic Study of the Neonatal Brain, 435

    Neonatal Brain Study, 437

PART **VII** **Vascular System,** 446

SECTION ONE ▪ Image Protocols for Abdominal Doppler and Color Flow Studies, 446

    Mesenteric Arterial Study, 448
    Renal Arterial Study, 453
    Examples of Various Venous Blood Flow Patterns and Duplex Protocols, 460
    Image Examples of Various Studies, 464

SECTION TWO ▪ Image Protocol for Cerebrovascular Duplex Scanning, 467

    Cerebrovascular Study, 469

SECTION THREE ▪ Image Protocols for Peripheral Arterial and Venous Duplex Scanning, 480

    Lower Limb Arterial Duplex Study, 482
    Lower Limb Venous Duplex Study, 498

PART **VIII** **Echocardiography,** 508

SECTION ONE ▪ Image Protocol for the Sonographic Study of the Adult Heart, 508

    Adult Heart Study, 509

SECTION TWO ▪ Image Protocol for the Sonographic Study of the Pediatric Heart, 540

    Pediatric Heart Study, 541

PART **IX** **Abbreviation Glossary,** 556

INTRODUCTION:
PURPOSE AND USE

Pocket Protocols is a response to the need for a practical imaging reference to use during ultrasound examinations.

The majority of the image protocols follow the American Institute of Ultrasound in Medicine's (AIUM) imaging guidelines. Any other image protocols are patterned after the AIUM's suggestions and the authors' collective experiences.

Pocket Protocols is a reference devoted to documenting technically accurate and thorough ultrasound image studies for diagnostic interpretation by the physician. These comprehensive imaging protocols include image and labeling examples for abdominal, pelvic, obstetric, small parts, vascular, and echocardiography studies.

Images are presented in a logical manner and specify the scanning plane and area of interest.

These reference materials are just that. They do not include or endorse the exclusion of the necessary prerequisites for accomplished scanning skills.

I hope *Pocket Protocols* serve as a practical reference and imaging standard that helps sonographers obtain comprehensive, consistent, and technically accurate image representations of ultrasound studies.

Betty Bates Tempkin, BA, RT(R), RDMS

IMAGE PROTOCOL FOR ABNORMAL SONOGRAPHIC FINDINGS

This section describes a universal imaging protocol for documenting pathology, regardless of the type. All pathology visualized by ultrasound in some way disrupts the normal sonographic pattern of the organ or structure involved and may alter its shape, size, contour, position, or textural appearance. Although familiarity with specific diseases and abnormalities is not necessary to document them accurately for physician interpretation, an understanding of pathological processes and the ways in which they affect interdependent body systems can be beneficial.

Criteria for Documenting Abnormal Sonographic Findings

- Survey of the abnormality in at least 2 scanning planes following the survey of the primary area(s) of interest. (This is not to say that the abnormality is not evaluated as the area of interest is evaluated, but it ensures that a total evaluation is made of a structure, not just its abnormal part.)
- Volume measurement of the abnormality.
- High- and low-gain technical setting images of the abnormality in at least 2 scanning planes.

Required Images

1. Longitudinal image of the abnormality *with measurement from the most superior to most inferior margin.*

   Labeled: **"ORGAN or STRUCTURE" or "SITE LOCATION" and "SCANNING PLANE"**

SCANNING TIP: Required images of abnormal findings follow the study's required images of the area(s) of interest.

SCANNING TIP: In cases where the origin of an abnormality cannot be determined, adjacent structures must be noted for a site location. Look for bright, echogenic interfaces where fat separates adjacent structures.

---

2. Same image as number 1, *without measurement calipers.*

   Labeled: **"ORGAN or STRUCTURE" or "SITE LOCATION" and "SCANNING PLANE"**

3. Axial image of the abnormality *with measurement from the most anterior to most posterior margin and from the most lateral to lateral or lateral to medial margin.*

   Labeled: **"ORGAN or STRUCTURE" or "SITE LOCATION" and "SCANNING PLANE"**

4. Same image as number 3, *without measurement calipers.*

   Labeled: **"ORGAN or STRUCTURE" or "SITE LOCATION" and "SCANNING PLANE"**

5. Longitudinal image of the abnormality with high-gain technique.

   Labeled: **"ORGAN or STRUCTURE" or "SITE LOCATION" and "SCANNING PLANE," HIGH GAIN**

6. Axial image of the abnormality with high-gain technique.

   Labeled: **"ORGAN or STRUCTURE" or "SITE LOCATION" and "SCANNING PLANE," HIGH GAIN**

7. Longitudinal image of the abnormality with low-gain technique.

   Labeled: **"ORGAN or STRUCTURE" or "SITE LOCATION" and "SCANNING PLANE," LOW GAIN**

8. Axial image of the abnormality with low-gain technique.

   Labeled: **"ORGAN or STRUCTURE" or "SITE LOCATION" and "SCANNING PLANE," LOW GAIN**

PART II

THE ABDOMEN

SECTION ONE ▪ Image Protocols for Full Sonographic Studies of the Abdomen

This section includes extensive images of the area(s) of interest accompanied by limited views of other major abdominal structures.

- Liver Study With Full Abdomen
- Aorta Study With Full Abdomen
- Inferior Vena Cava Study With Full Abdomen
- Gallbladder and Biliary Tract Study With Full Abdomen
- Pancreas Study With Full Abdomen
- Renal Study With Full Abdomen
- Spleen Study With Full Abdomen

Criteria

- Begin studies with a survey of abdominal structures in at least 2 scanning planes.
- Do not share study results with the patient. Legally, only physicians can give diagnoses.

Liver Study With Full Abdomen

Liver • Longitudinal Images

1. Longitudinal image of the left lobe of the liver to include the inferior margin and the aorta.

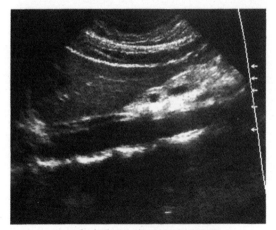

Labeled: **LIVER SAG LT LOBE**

2. Longitudinal image of the left lobe of the liver to include the diaphragm and caudate lobe.

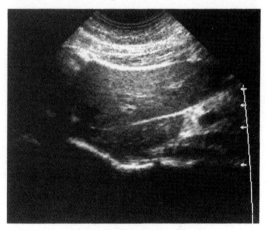

Labeled: **LIVER SAG LT LOBE**

3. Longitudinal image of the right lobe of the liver to include the inferior vena cava (IVC) where it passes through the liver.

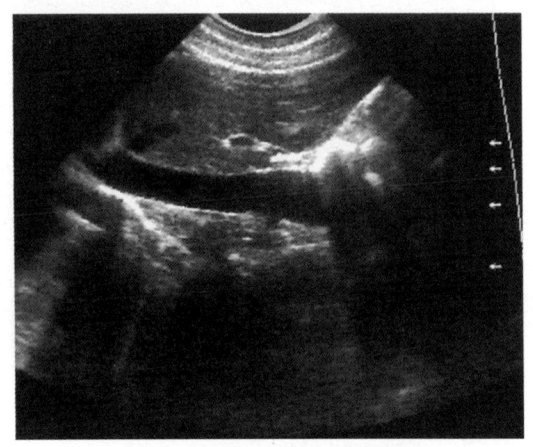

Labeled: **LIVER SAG RT LOBE**

4. Longitudinal image of the right lobe of the liver to include the main lobar fissure, gallbladder, and portal vein.

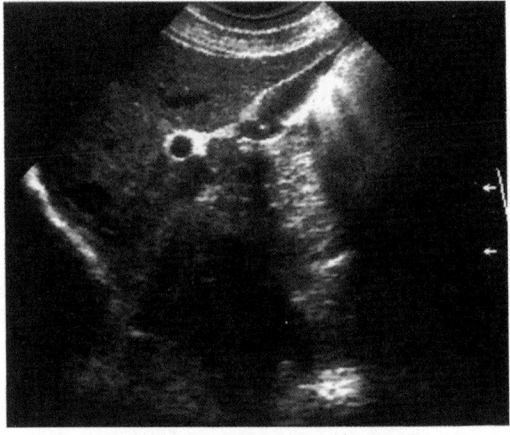

Labeled: **LIVER SAG RT LOBE**

5. Longitudinal image of the right lobe of the liver to include part of the right kidney for parenchyma comparison.

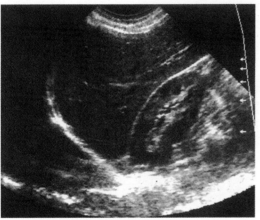

Labeled: **LIVER SAG RT LOBE**

6. Longitudinal image of the right lobe of the liver to include the dome and adjacent pleural space.

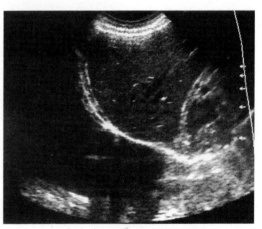

Labeled: **LIVER SAG RT LOBE**

PART III

Liver • Axial Images

7. Axial image of the left lobe of the liver to include its lateral margin.

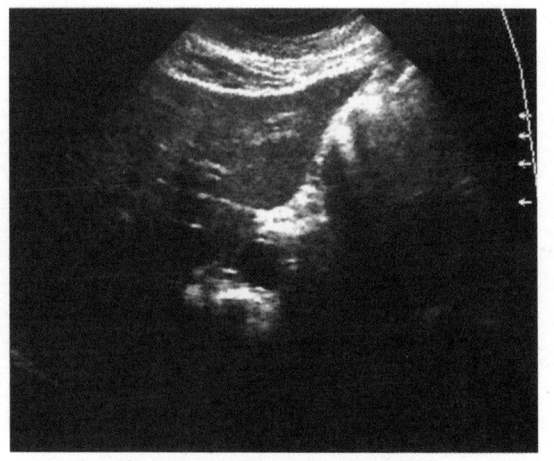

Labeled: **LIVER TRV LT LOBE**

8. Axial image of the left lobe of the liver to include the ligamentum teres.

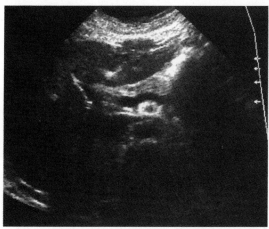

Labeled: **LIVER TRV LT LOBE**

SCANNING TIP: Depending on liver size and shape, it may be possible to document an axial image of the left lobe that includes both the lateral margin and ligamentum teres. If so, label the image as follows:
LIVER TRV LT LOBE

9. Axial image of the right lobe of the liver to include the hepatic veins.

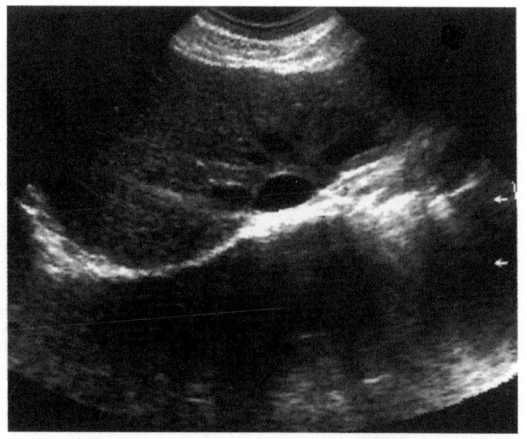

Labeled: **LIVER TRV RT LOBE**

10. Axial image of the right lobe of the liver to include the right and left branches of the portal vein.

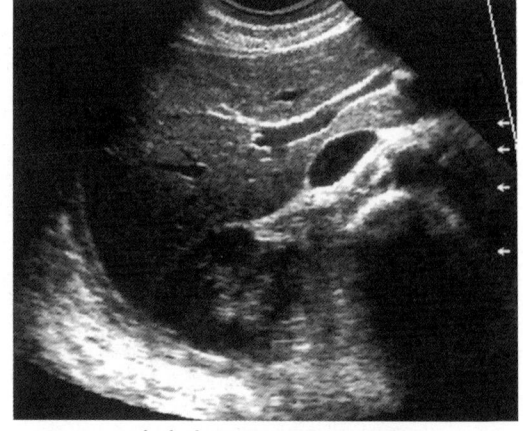

Labeled: **LIVER TRV RT LOBE**

11. Axial image of the right lobe of the liver to include the right lateral inferior lobe.

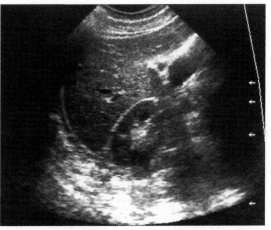

Labeled: **LIVER TRV RT LOBE**

PART III

12. Axial image of the right lobe of the liver to include the dome and adjacent pleural space.

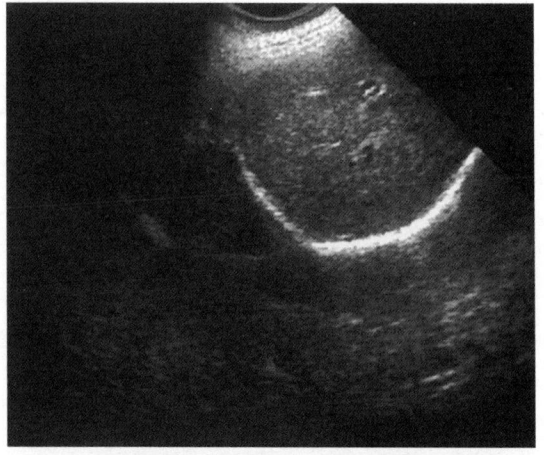

Labeled: **LIVER TRV RT LOBE**

SCANNING TIP: Routine measurements of the liver are not required.

Aorta • Longitudinal Image

SCANNING TIP: The images of the aorta may be included with the liver images if the aorta is well visualized.

13. Longitudinal image of the proximal and middle aorta.

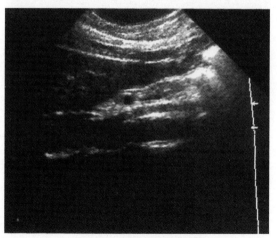

Labeled: **AORTA SAG MID**

Aorta • Axial Image

14. Axial image of the middle aorta at the level of the renal arteries.

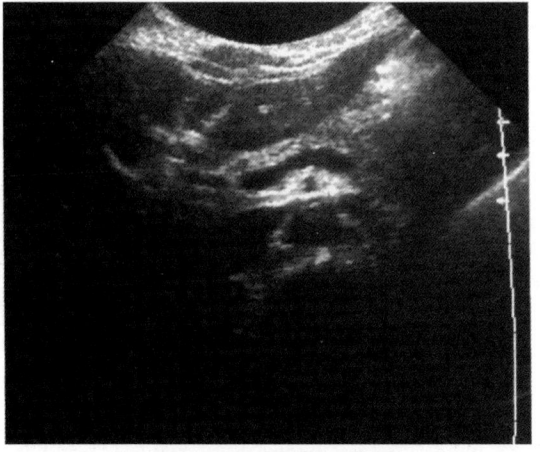

Labeled: **AORTA TRV MID**

Inferior Vena Cava • Longitudinal Image

SCANNING TIP: The images of the IVC may be included with the liver images if the IVC is well visualized.

15. Longitudinal image of the distal and middle IVC.

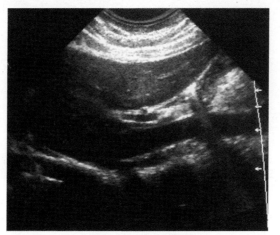

Labeled: **IVC SAG DISTAL**

PART III

Inferior Vena Cava • Axial Image

16. Axial image of the distal IVC to include the hepatic veins.

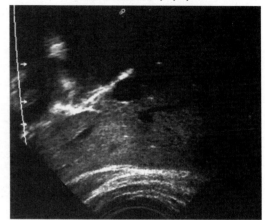

Labeled: **IVC TRV DISTAL**

Gallbladder • Longitudinal Image

17. Long axis image of the gallbladder.

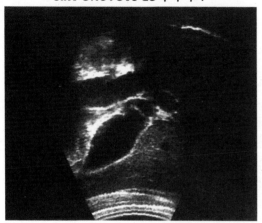

Labeled: **GB SAG LONG AXIS**

Gallbladder • Axial Image

18. Axial image of the gallbladder fundus.

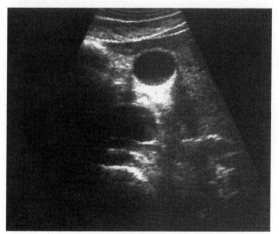

Labeled: **GB TRV FUNDUS**

Biliary Tract • Longitudinal Images

19. Longitudinal image of the common hepatic duct (CHD).

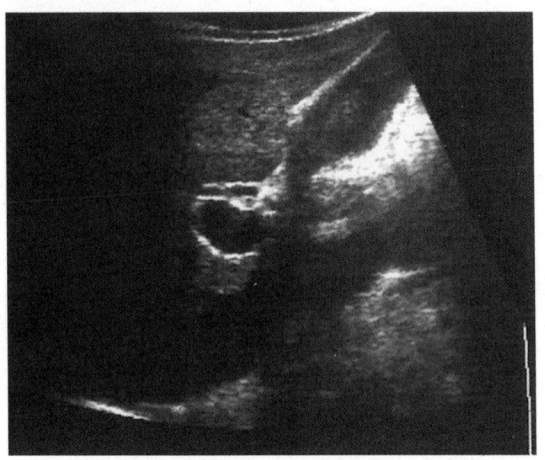

Labeled: **SAG CHD**

SCANNING TIP: Biliary tract images may be magnified to aid interpretation.

SCANNING TIP: The CHD image may be omitted if the CHD was visualized on the gallbladder long axis image.

20. Longitudinal image of the common bile duct *with anterior to posterior measurement at the widest margins of the lumen.*

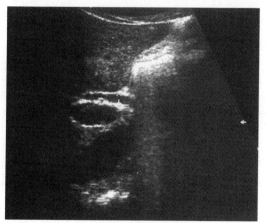

Labeled: **SAG CBD**

21. Same image as number 20 *without measurement calipers.*

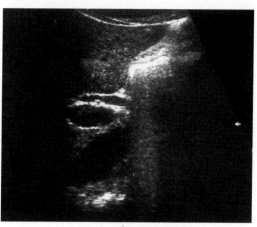

Labeled: **SAG CBD**

Pancreas • Longitudinal Images

22. Long axis image of the pancreas to include as much head, uncinate, neck, body, tail, and pancreatic duct as possible.

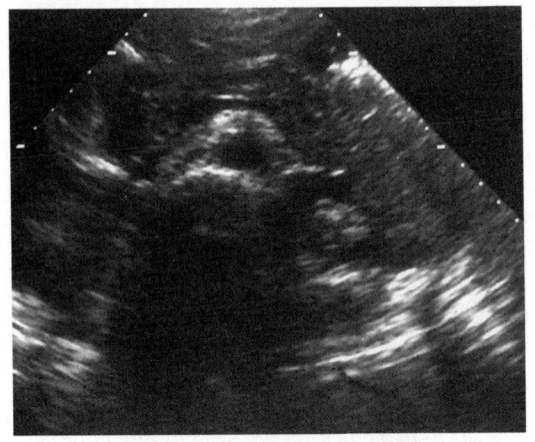

Labeled: **PANC TRV LONG AXIS**

23. Longitudinal image of the pancreas head to include the uncinate process and common bile duct (if bile filled).

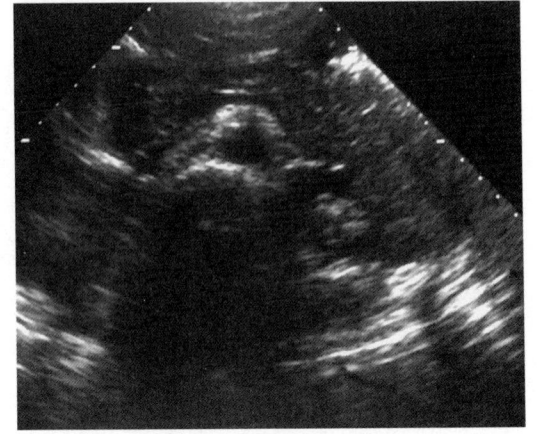

Labeled: **PANC TRV HEAD**

Pancreas • Axial Image

24. Axial image of the pancreas head to include the common bile duct (if bile filled).

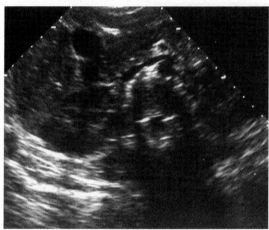

Labeled: **PANC SAG HEAD**

SCANNING TIP: In some cases, a portion or all of the pancreas cannot be visualized because of overlying bowel gas and the patient cannot be given fluids to displace the gas. When this occurs, and every effort has been made to image the pancreas, take the required images in the designated areas and add "AREA" to the labeling.

Right Kidney • Longitudinal Image

25. Long axis image of the right kidney.

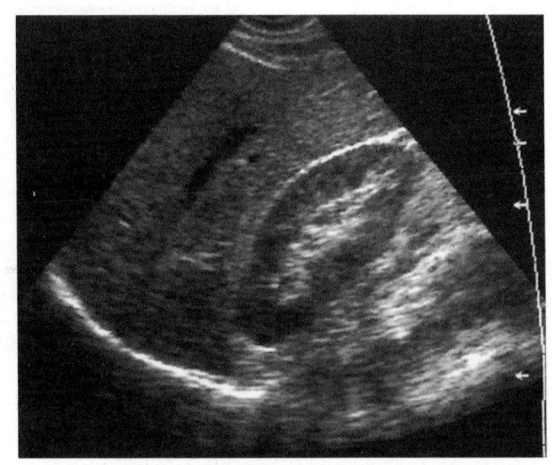

Labeled: **RT KID SAG LONG AXIS**

SCANNING TIP: Take an additional image of the superior and/or inferior poles if they are not clearly represented on the long axis image. Label accordingly.

Right Kidney • Axial Image

26. Axial image of the right kidney midportion to include the hilum.

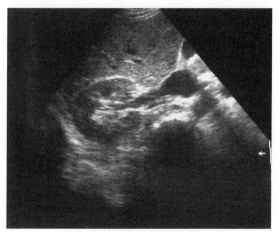

Labeled: **RT KID TRV MID**

PART III

Left Kidney • Longitudinal Image

27. Long axis image of the left kidney.

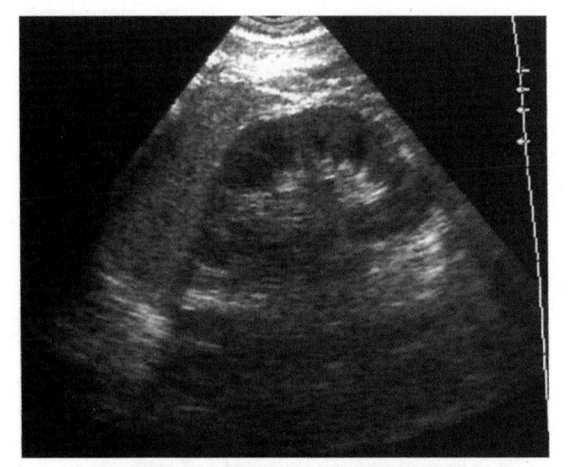

Labeled: **LT KID COR LONG AXIS**

SCANNING TIP: Take an additional image of the superior and/or inferior poles if they are not clearly represented on the long axis image. Label accordingly.

Left Kidney • Axial Image

28. Axial image of the left kidney midportion to include the hilum.

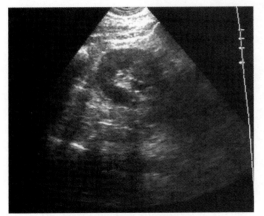

Labeled: **LT KID LT TRV MID**

Spleen • Longitudinal Image

29. Long axis or longitudinal image of the spleen to include the adjacent pleural space superiorly and portion of the left kidney inferiorly.

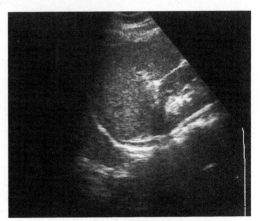

Labeled: **SPLEEN COR LONG AXIS or SPLEEN COR**

PART III

Spleen • Axial Image

30. Axial image of the spleen to include the anterior and posterior margins.

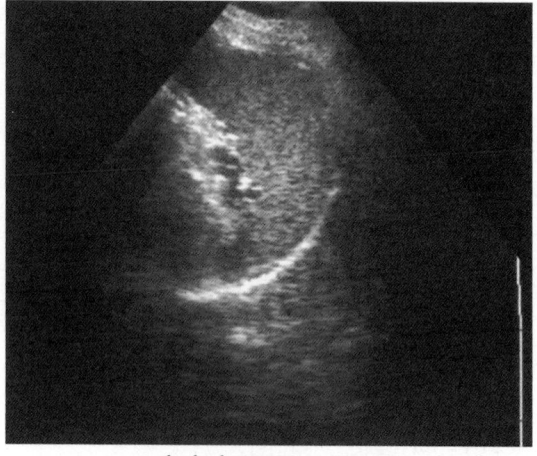

Labeled: **SPLEEN LT TRV**

Aorta Study With Full Abdomen

Liver • Longitudinal Images

1. Longitudinal image of the left lobe of the liver to include the inferior margin and the aorta.

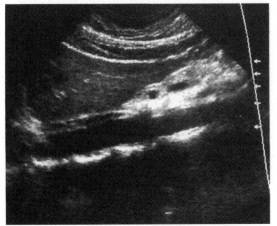

Labeled: **LIVER SAG LT LOBE**

2. Longitudinal image of the left lobe of the liver to include the diaphragm and caudate lobe.

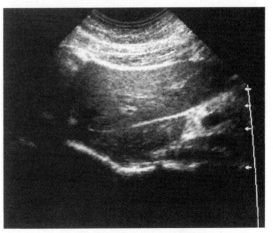

Labeled: **LIVER SAG LT LOBE**

PART III

3. Longitudinal image of the right lobe of the liver to include the IVC where it passes through the liver.

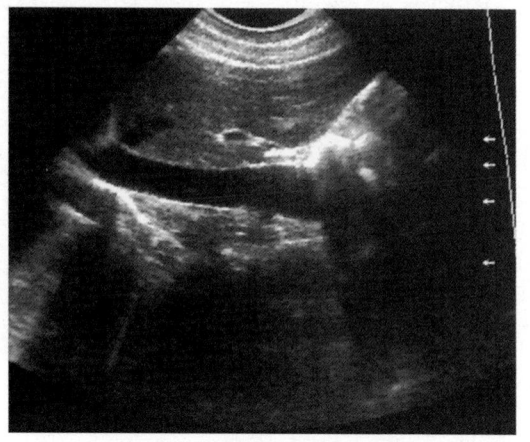

Labeled: **LIVER SAG RT LOBE**

4. Longitudinal image of the right lobe of the liver to include the main lobar fissure, gallbladder, and portal vein.

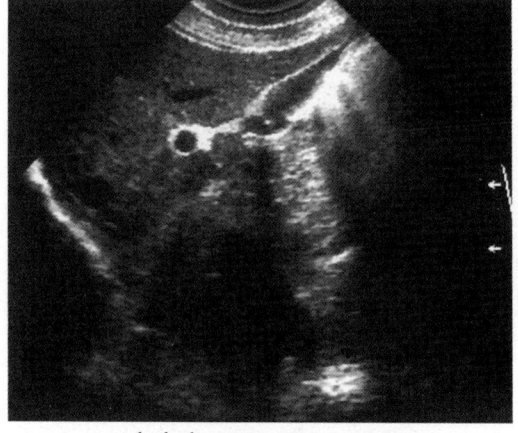

Labeled: **LIVER SAG RT LOBE**

5. Longitudinal image of the right lobe of the liver to include part of the right kidney for parenchyma comparison.

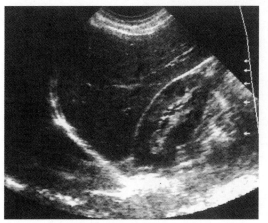

Labeled: **LIVER SAG RT LOBE**

6. Longitudinal image of the right lobe of the liver to include the dome and adjacent pleural space.

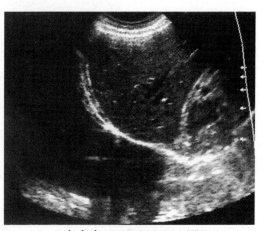

Labeled: **LIVER SAG RT LOBE**

PART III

Liver • Axial Images

7. Axial image of the left lobe of the liver to include its lateral margin.

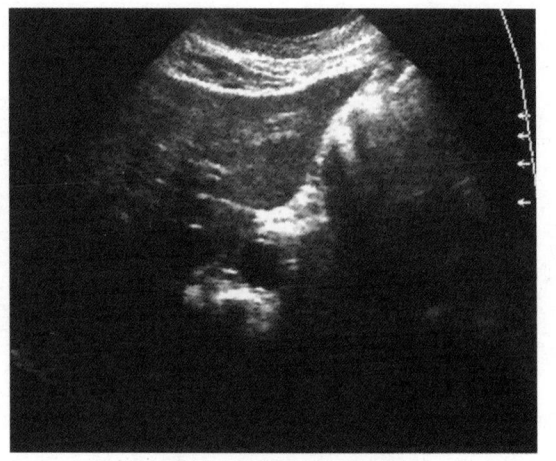

Labeled: **LIVER TRV LT LOBE**

8. Axial image of the left lobe of the liver to include the ligamentum teres.

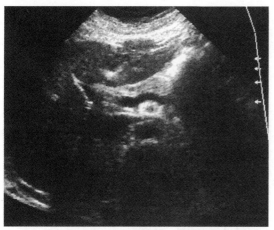

Labeled: **LIVER TRV LT LOBE**

SCANNING TIP: Depending on liver size and shape, it may be possible to document an axial image of the left lobe that includes both the lateral margin and ligamentum teres. If so, label the image as follows:
LIVER TRV LT LOBE

9. Axial image of the right lobe of the liver to include the hepatic veins.

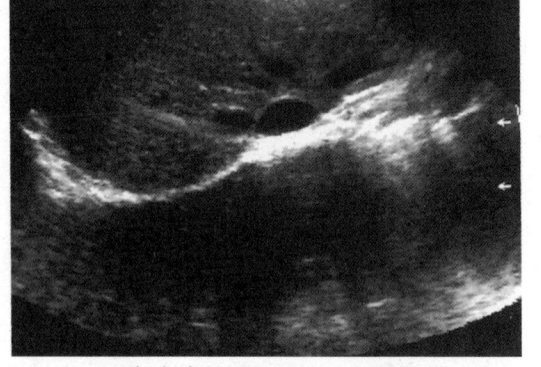

Labeled: **LIVER TRV RT LOBE**

10. Axial image of the right lobe of the liver to include the right and left branches of the portal vein.

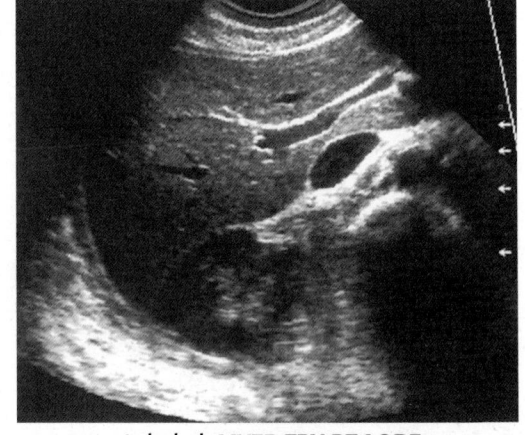

Labeled: **LIVER TRV RT LOBE**

11. Axial image of the right lobe of the liver to include the right lateral inferior lobe.

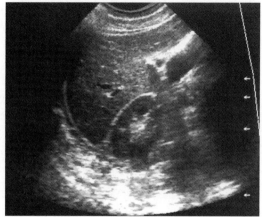

Labeled: **LIVER TRV RT LOBE**

12. Axial image of the right lobe of the liver to include the dome and adjacent pleural space.

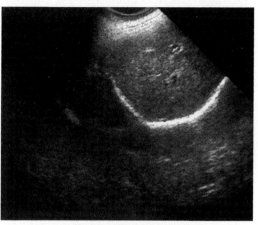

Labeled: **LIVER TRV RT LOBE**

Aorta • Longitudinal Images

13. Longitudinal image of the proximal aorta (inferior to the diaphragm, superior to the celiac trunk).

14. Longitudinal image of the middle aorta (inferior to the celiac trunk along the length of the superior mesenteric artery).

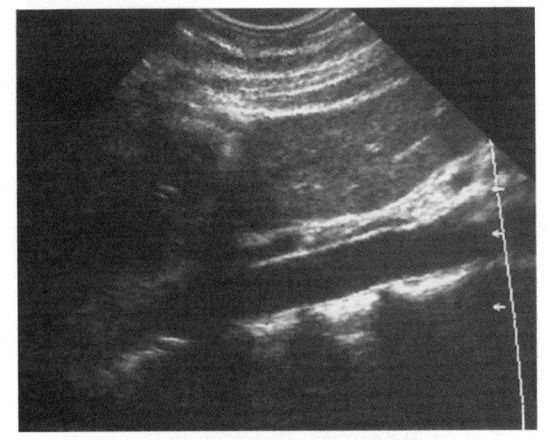

Labeled: **AORTA SAG PROX**

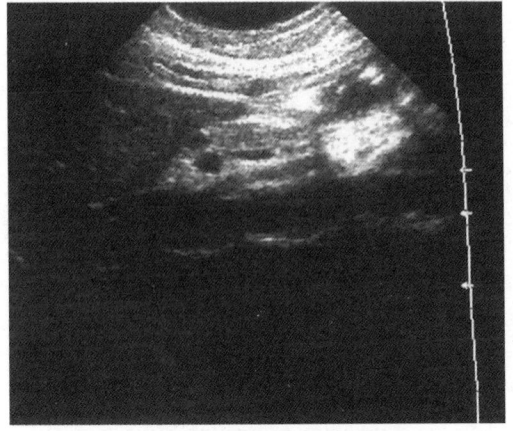

Labeled: **AORTA SAG MID**

15. Longitudinal image of the distal aorta (inferior to the superior mesenteric artery, superior to the bifurcation).

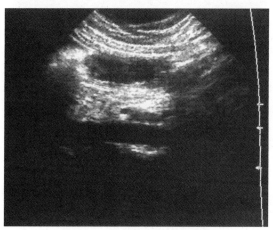

Labeled: **AORTA SAG DISTAL**

16. Longitudinal image of the aorta bifurcation (common iliac arteries).

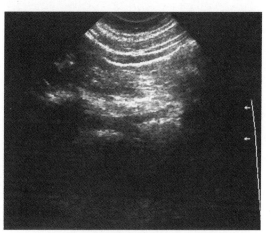

Labeled: **AORTA SAG BIF RT or LT OBL or AORTA LT COR BIF**

Aorta • Axial Images

17. Axial image of the proximal aorta (inferior to the diaphragm, superior to the celiac trunk) *with anterior to posterior measurement* (calipers outside wall to outside wall).

18. Same image as number 17 *without measurement calipers*.

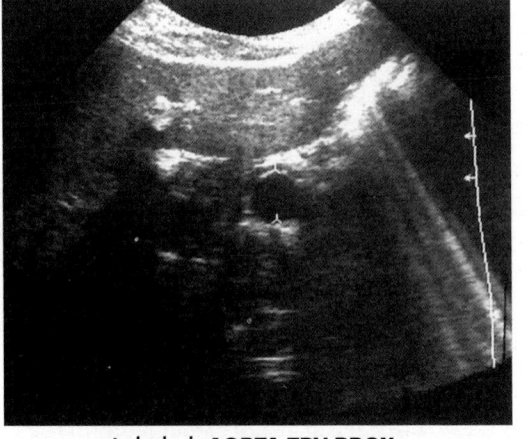

Labeled: **AORTA TRV PROX**

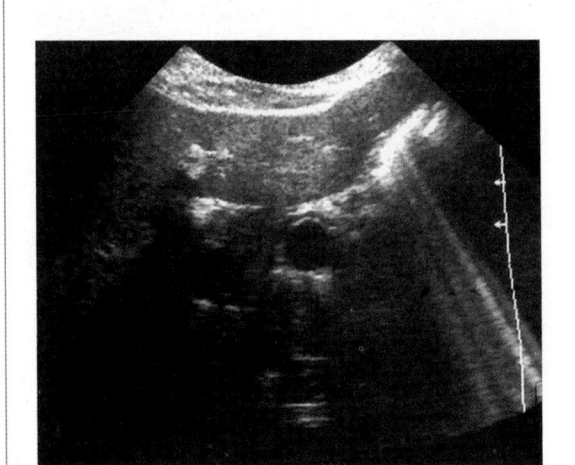

Labeled: **AORTA TRV PROX**

19. Axial image of the middle aorta (inferior to the celiac trunk along the length of the superior mesenteric artery) *with anterior to posterior measurement* (calipers outside wall to outside wall).

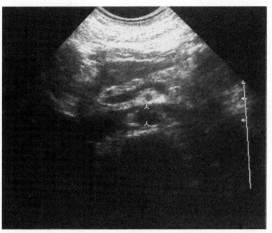

Labeled: **AORTA TRV MID**

20. Same image as number 19, *without measurement calipers.*

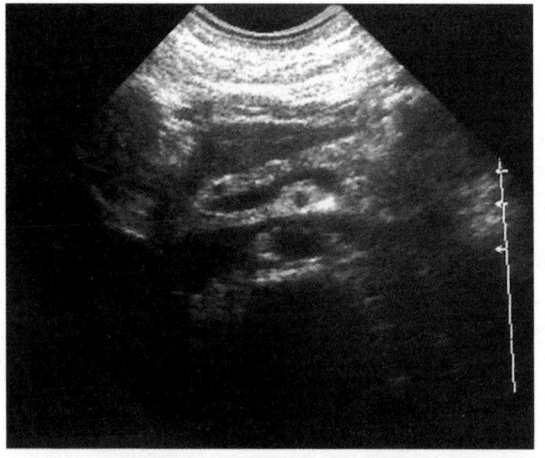

Labeled: **AORTA TRV MID**

SCANNING TIP: If the renal arteries were represented on number 19, numbers 21 and/or 22 may be omitted.

21. Longitudinal image of the right renal artery.

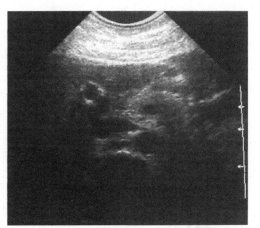

Labeled: **RT RENAL ART TRV**

22. Longitudinal image of the left renal artery.

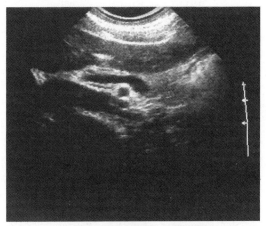

Labeled: **LT RENAL ART TRV**

PART III

23. Axial image of the distal aorta (inferior to the superior mesenteric artery, superior to the bifurcation) *with anterior to posterior measurement* (calipers outside wall to outside wall).

24. Same image as number 23, *without measurement calipers.*

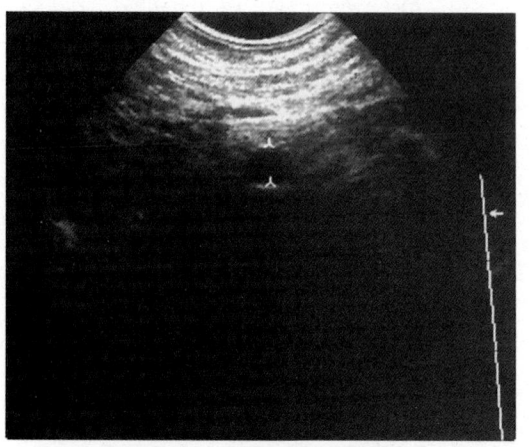

Labeled: **AORTA TRV DISTAL**

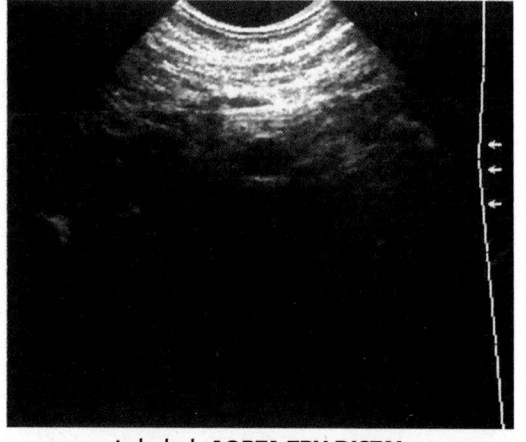

Labeled: **AORTA TRV DISTAL**

25. Axial image of aorta bifurcation (common iliac arteries).

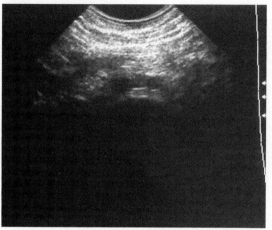

Labeled: **AORTA TRV BIF**

Inferior Vena Cava • Longitudinal Image

> **SCANNING TIP:** The images of the IVC may be included with the liver images if the IVC is well visualized.

26. Longitudinal image of the distal and middle IVC.

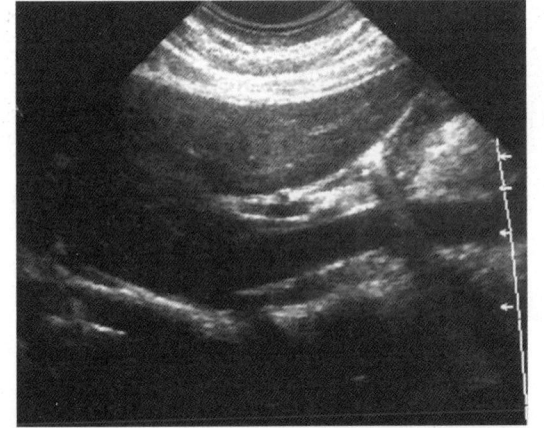

Labeled: **IVC SAG DISTAL**

Inferior Vena Cava • Axial Image

27. Axial image of the distal IVC to include the hepatic veins.

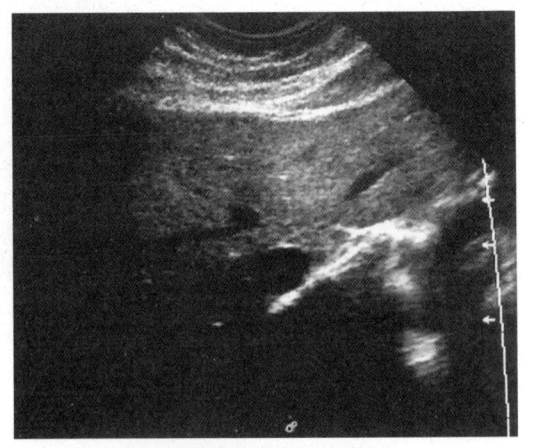

Labeled: **IVC TRV DISTAL**

Gallbladder • Longitudinal Image

28. Long axis image of the gallbladder.

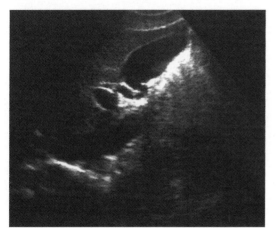

Labeled: **GB SAG LONG AXIS**

Gallbladder • Axial Image

29. Axial image of the gallbladder fundus.

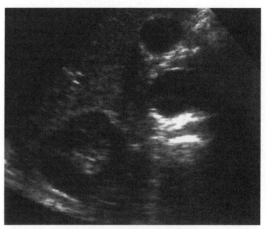

Labeled: **GB TRV FUNDUS**

PART III

Biliary Tract • Longitudinal Images

> **SCANNING TIP:** Biliary tract images may be magnified to aid interpretation.
>
> **SCANNING TIP:** The CHD image may be omitted if the CHD was visualized on the gallbladder long axis image.

30. Longitudinal image of the CHD.

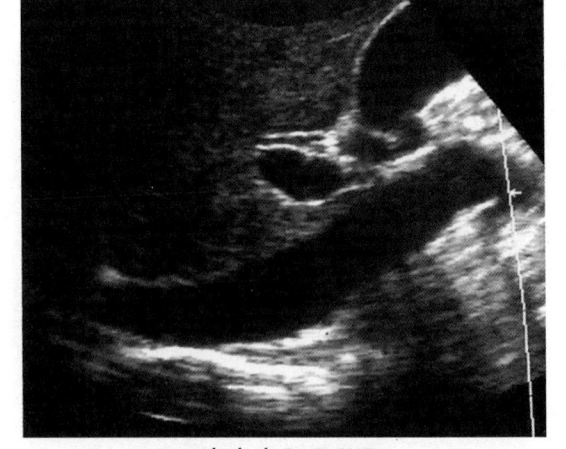

Labeled: **SAG CHD**

31. Longitudinal image of the common bile duct *with anterior to posterior measurement at the widest margins of the lumen.*

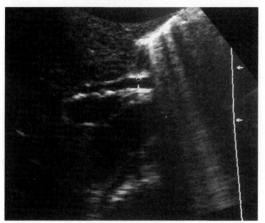

Labeled: **SAG CBD**

32. Same image as number 31 *without measurement calipers.*

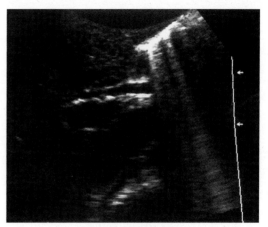

Labeled: **SAG CBD**

PART III

Pancreas • Longitudinal Images

33. Long axis image of the pancreas to include as much head, uncinate, neck, body, tail, and pancreatic duct as possible.

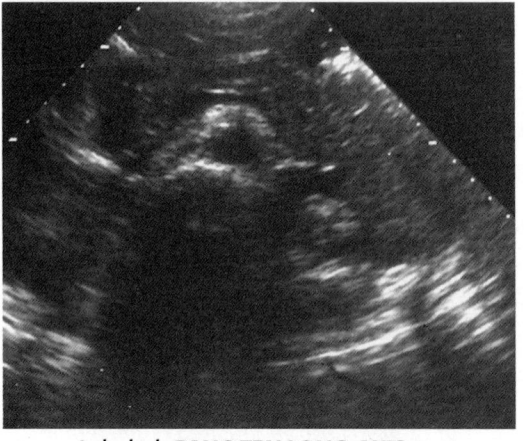

Labeled: **PANC TRV LONG AXIS**

34. Longitudinal image of the pancreas head to include the uncinate process and common bile duct (if bile filled).

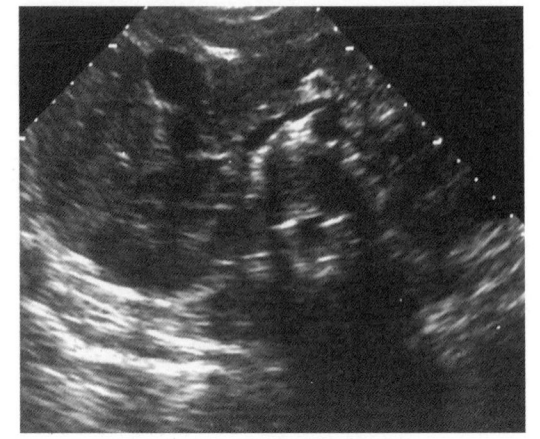

Labeled: **PANC TRV HEAD**

Pancreas • Axial Image

35. Axial image of the pancreas head to include the common bile duct (if bile filled).

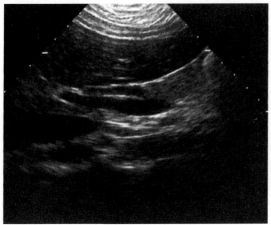

Labeled: **PANC SAG HEAD**

> **SCANNING TIP:** In some cases, a portion or all of the pancreas cannot be visualized because of overlying bowel gas and the patient cannot be given fluids to displace the gas. When this occurs, and every effort has been made to image the pancreas, take the required images in the designated areas and add "AREA" to the labeling.

PART III

Right Kidney • Longitudinal Image

36. Long axis image of the right kidney.

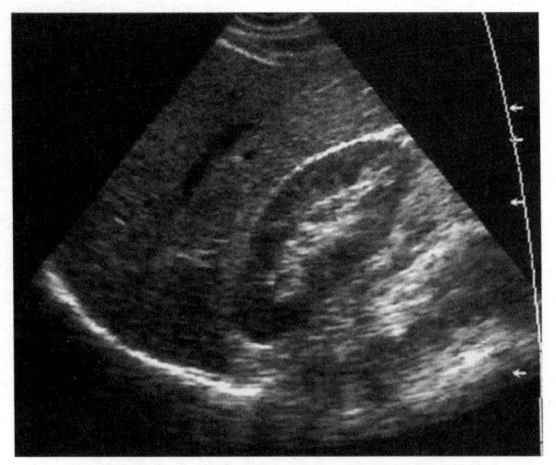

Labeled: **RT KID SAG LONG AXIS**

SCANNING TIP: Take an additional image of the superior and/or inferior poles if they are not clearly represented on the long axis image. Label accordingly.

Right Kidney • Axial Image

37. Axial image of the right kidney midportion to include the hilum.

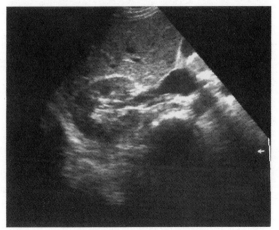

Labeled: **RT KID TRV MID**

Left Kidney • Longitudinal Image

38. Long axis image of the left kidney.

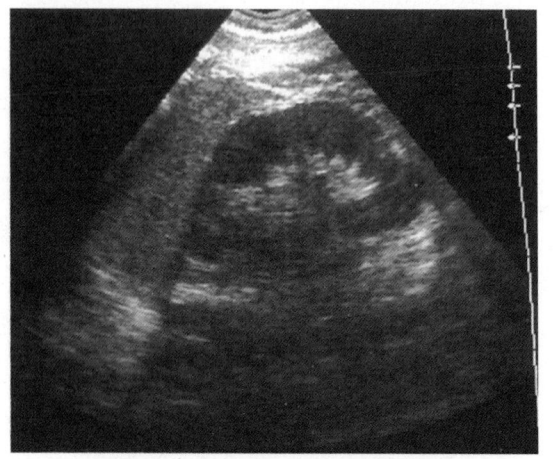

Labeled: **LT KID COR LONG AXIS**

SCANNING TIP: Take an additional image of the superior and/or inferior poles if they are not clearly represented on the long axis image. Label accordingly.

Left Kidney • Axial Image

39. Axial image of the left kidney midportion to include the hilum.

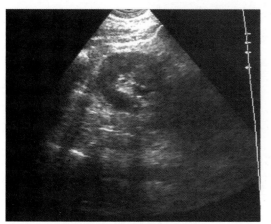

Labeled: **LT KID LT TRV MID**

Spleen • Longitudinal Image

40. Long axis or longitudinal image of the spleen to include the adjacent pleural space superiorly and a portion of the left kidney inferiorly.

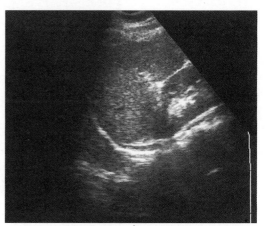

Labeled: **SPLEEN COR LONG AXIS or SPLEEN COR**

PART III

Spleen • Axial Image

41. Axial image of the spleen to include the anterior and posterior margins.

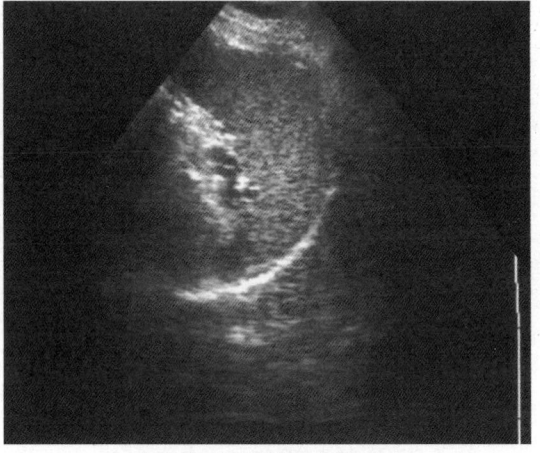

Labeled: **SPLEEN LT TRV**

Inferior Vena Cava Study With Full Abdomen

Liver • Longitudinal Images

1. Longitudinal image of the left lobe of the liver to include the inferior margin and the aorta.

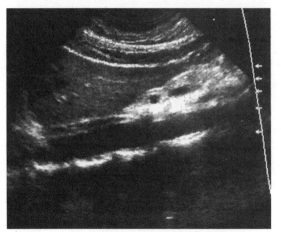

Labeled: **LIVER TRV LT LOBE**

2. Longitudinal image of the left lobe of the liver to include the diaphragm and caudate lobe.

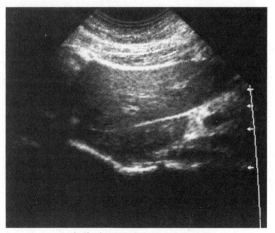

Labeled: **LIVER SAG LT LOBE**

3. Longitudinal image of the right lobe of the liver to include the IVC where it passes through the liver.

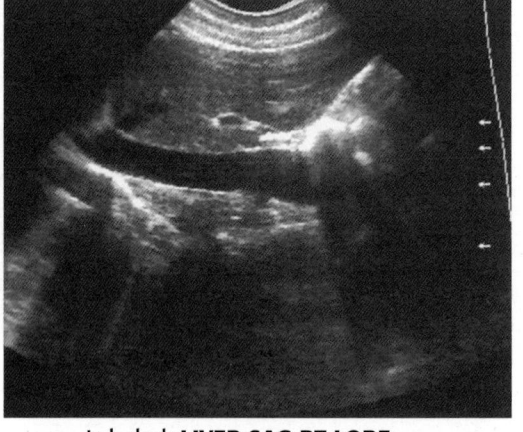

Labeled: **LIVER SAG RT LOBE**

4. Longitudinal image of the right lobe of the liver to include the main lobar fissure, gallbladder, and portal vein.

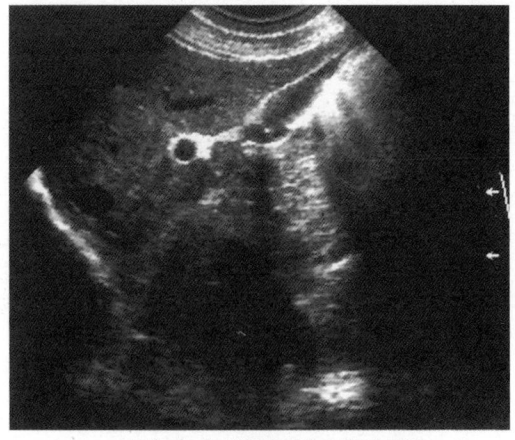

Labeled: **LIVER SAG RT LOBE**

5. Longitudinal image of the right lobe of the liver to include part of the right kidney for parenchyma comparison.

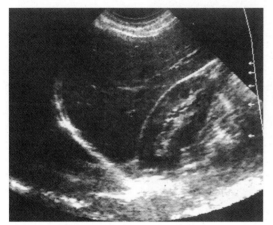

Labeled: **LIVER SAG RT LOBE**

6. Longitudinal image of the right lobe of the liver to include the dome and adjacent pleural space.

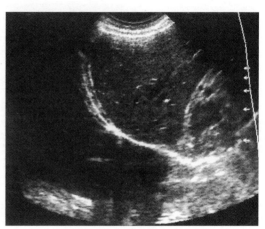

Labeled: **LIVER SAG RT LOBE**

Liver • Axial Images

7. Axial image of the left lobe of the liver to include its lateral margin.

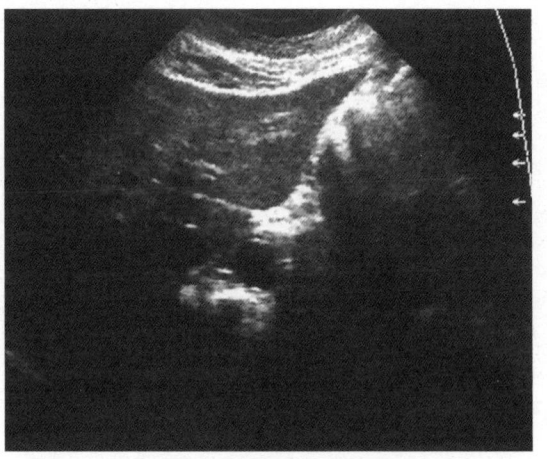

Labeled: **LIVER TRV LT LOBE**

8. Axial image of the left lobe of the liver to include the ligamentum teres.

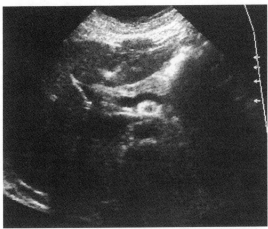

Labeled: **LIVER TRV RT LOBE**

SCANNING TIP: Depending on liver size and shape, it may be possible to document an axial image of the left lobe that includes both the lateral margin and ligamentum teres. If so, label the image as follows:
LIVER TRV LT LOBE

9. Axial image of the right lobe of the liver to include the hepatic veins.

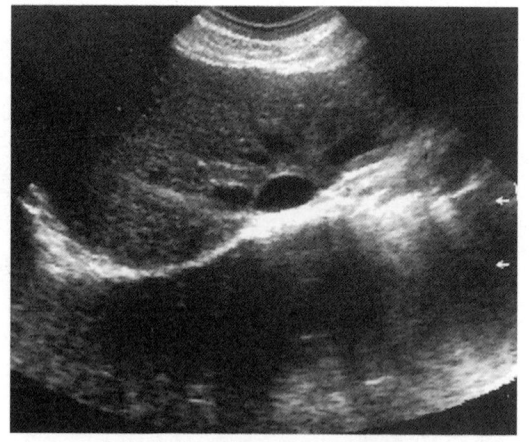

Labeled: **LIVER TRV RT LOBE**

10. Axial image of the right lobe of the liver to include the right and left branches of the portal vein.

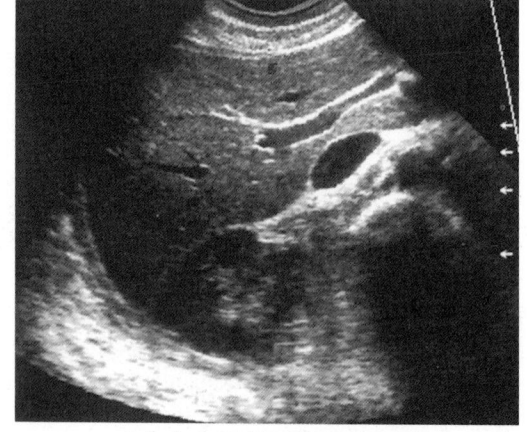

Labeled: **LIVER TRV RT LOBE**

11. Axial image of the right lobe of the liver to include the right lateral inferior lobe.

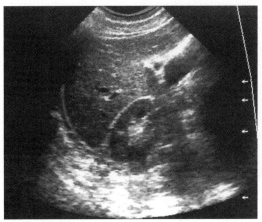

Labeled: **LIVER TRV RT LOBE**

12. Axial image of the right lobe of the liver to include the dome and adjacent pleural space.

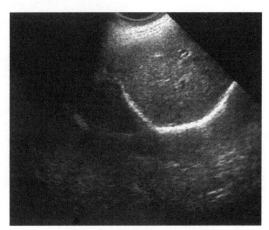

Labeled: **LIVER TRV RT LOBE**

Aorta • Longitudinal Image

SCANNING TIP: The images of the aorta may be included with the liver images if the aorta is well visualized.

13. Longitudinal image of the proximal and middle aorta.

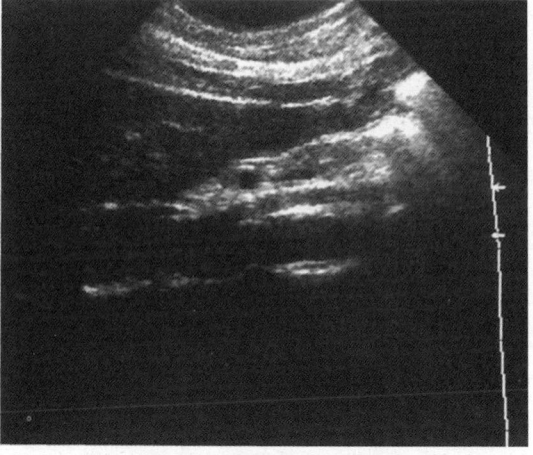

Labeled: **AORTA SAG MID**

Aorta • Axial Image

14. Axial image of the middle aorta at the level of the renal arteries.

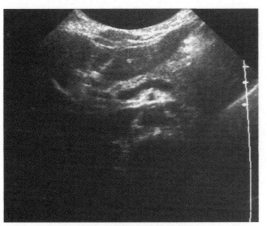

Labeled: **AORTA TRV MID**

Inferior Vena Cava • Longitudinal Images

15. Longitudinal image of the distal IVC to include the diaphragm and hepatic vein(s).

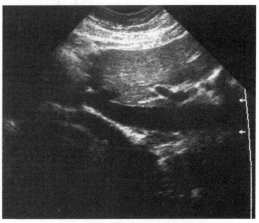

Labeled: **IVC SAG DISTAL**

PART III

16. Longitudinal image of the middle IVC at the level of the head of the pancreas.

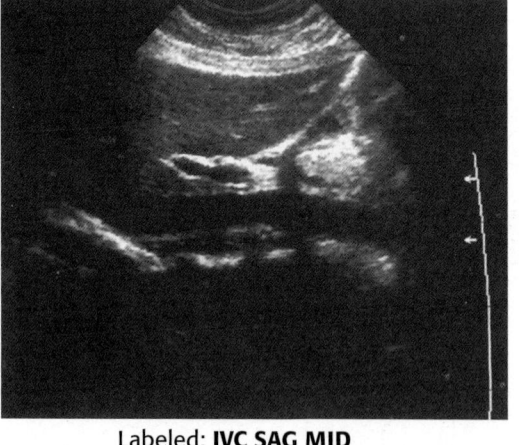

Labeled: **IVC SAG MID**

17. Longitudinal image of the proximal IVC.

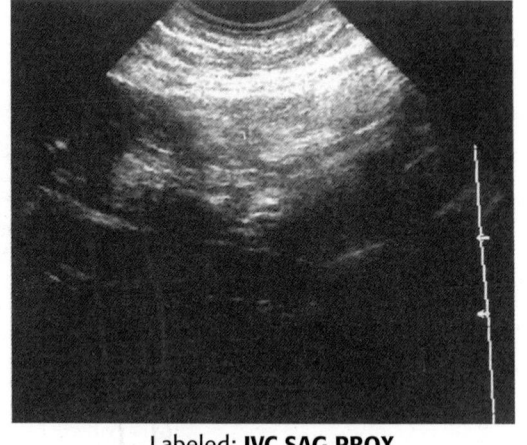

Labeled: **IVC SAG PROX**

18. Longitudinal image of the IVC bifurcation (common iliac veins).

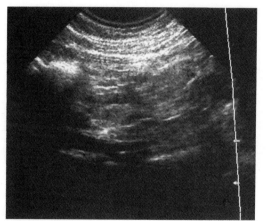

Labeled: **IVC SAG BIF RT or LT OBL or IVC SAG RT COR BIF**

Inferior Vena Cava • Axial Images

19. Axial image of the distal IVC to include the hepatic veins.

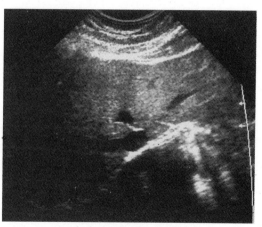

Labeled: **IVC TRV DISTAL**

20. Axial image of the IVC at the level of the renal veins.

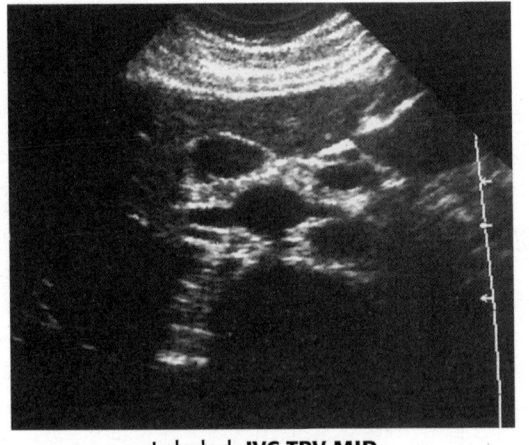

Labeled: **IVC TRV MID**

21. Axial image of the proximal IVC.

Labeled: **IVC TRV PROX**

22. Axial image of the IVC bifurcation (common iliac veins).

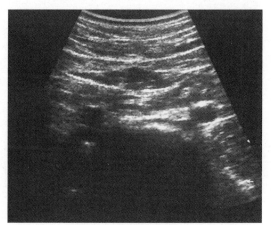

Labeled: **IVC TRV BIF**

Gallbladder • Longitudinal Image

23. Long axis image of the gallbladder.

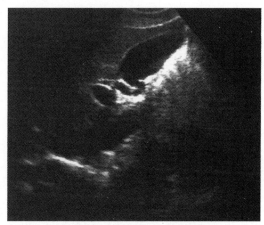

Labeled: **GB SAG LONG AXIS**

Gallbladder • Axial Image

24. Axial image of the gallbladder fundus.

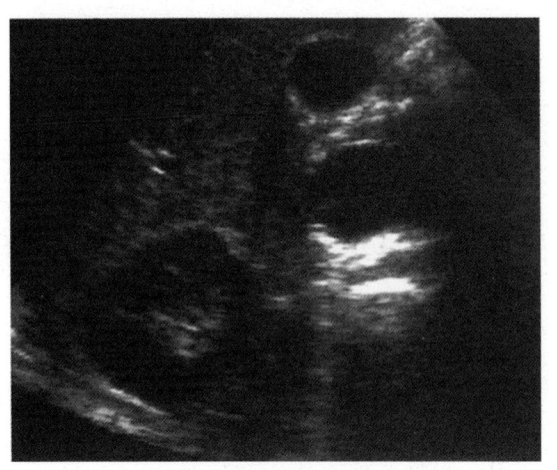

Labeled: **GB TRV FUNDUS**

Biliary Tract • Longitudinal Images

SCANNING TIP: Biliary tract images may be magnified to aid interpretation.

SCANNING TIP: The CHD image may be omitted if the CHD was visualized on the gallbladder long axis image.

25. Longitudinal image of the CHD.

26. Longitudinal image of the common bile duct *with anterior to posterior measurement at the widest margins of the lumen.*

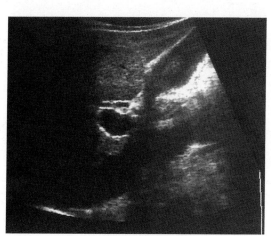

Labeled: **SAG CHD**

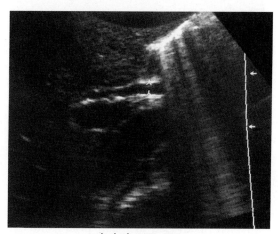

Labeled: **SAG CBD**

PART III

27. Same image as number 26 *without measurement calipers.*

Pancreas • Longitudinal Images

28. Long axis image of the pancreas to include as much head, uncinate, neck, body, tail, and pancreatic duct as possible.

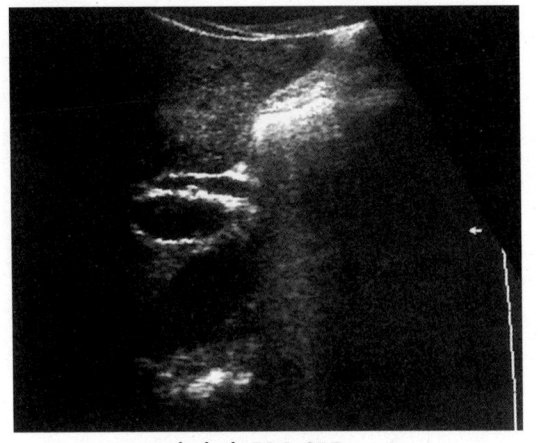

Labeled: **SAG CBD**

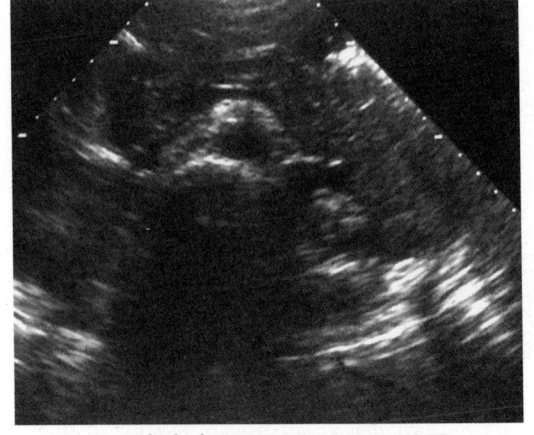

Labeled: **PANC TRV LONG AXIS**

29. Longitudinal image of the pancreas head to include the uncinate process and common bile duct (if bile filled).

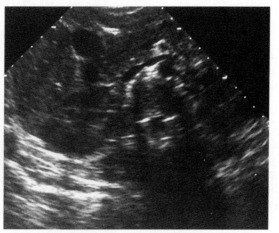

Labeled: **PANC TRV HEAD**

Pancreas • Axial Image

30. Axial image of the pancreas head to include the common bile duct (if bile filled).

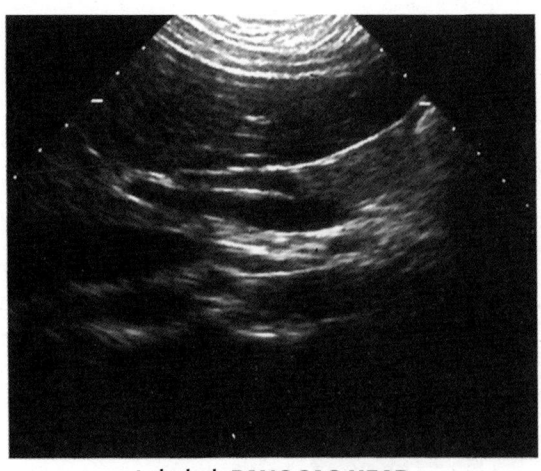

Labeled: **PANC SAG HEAD**

SCANNING TIP: In some cases, a portion or all of the pancreas cannot be visualized because of overlying bowel gas and the patient cannot be given fluids to displace the gas. When this occurs, and every effort has been made to image the pancreas, take the required images in the designated areas and add "AREA" to the labeling.

Right Kidney • Longitudinal Image

31. Long axis image of the right kidney.

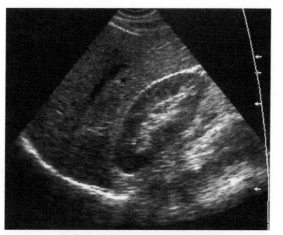

Labeled: **RT KID SAG LONG AXIS**

SCANNING TIP: Take an additional image of the superior and/or inferior poles if they are not clearly represented on the long axis image. Label accordingly.

Right Kidney • Axial Image

32. Axial image of the right kidney midportion to include the hilum.

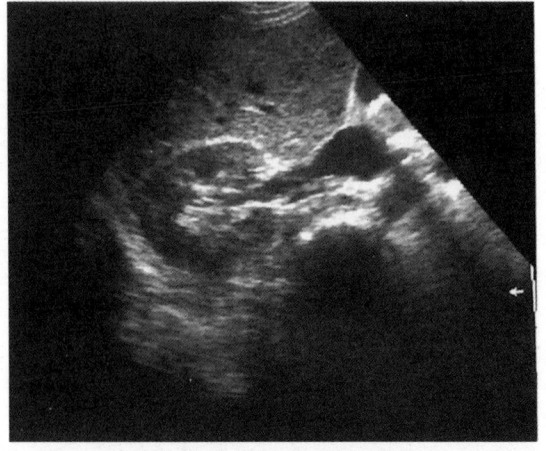

Labeled: **RT KID TRV MID**

Left Kidney • Longitudinal Image

33. Long axis image of the left kidney.

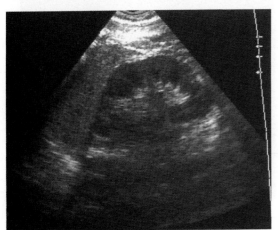

Labeled: **LT KID COR LONG AXIS**

SCANNING TIP: Take an additional image of the superior and/or inferior poles if they are not clearly represented on the long axis image. Label accordingly.

PART III

Left Kidney • Axial Image

34. Axial image of the left kidney midportion to include the hilum.

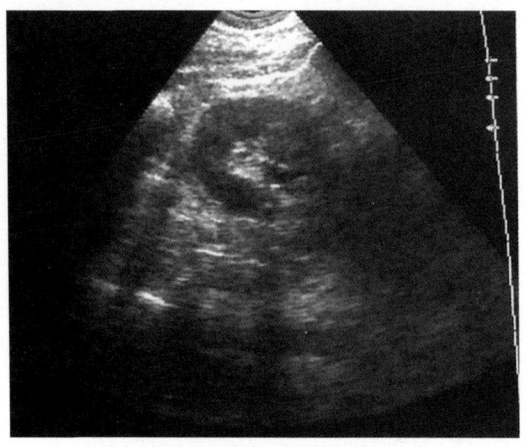

Labeled: **LT KID LT TRV MID**

Spleen • Longitudinal Image

35. Long axis or longitudinal image of the spleen to include the adjacent pleural space superiorly and portion of the left kidney inferiorly.

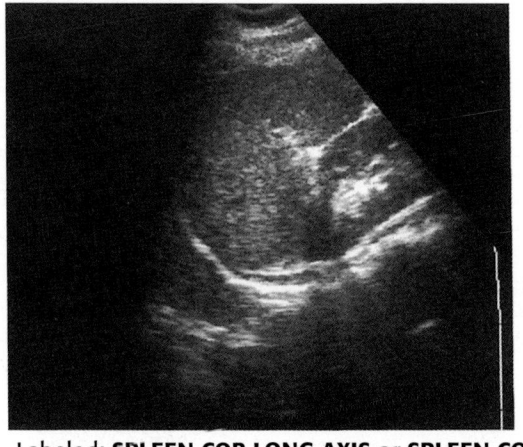

Labeled: **SPLEEN COR LONG AXIS or SPLEEN COR**

Spleen • Axial Image

36. Axial image of the spleen to include the anterior and posterior margins.

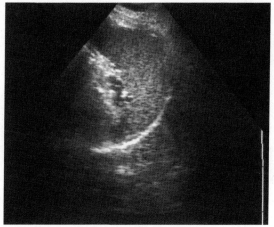

Labeled: **SPLEEN LT TRV**

Gallbladder and Biliary Tract Study With Full Abdomen

Liver • Longitudinal Images

1. Longitudinal image of the left lobe of the liver to include the inferior margin and the aorta.

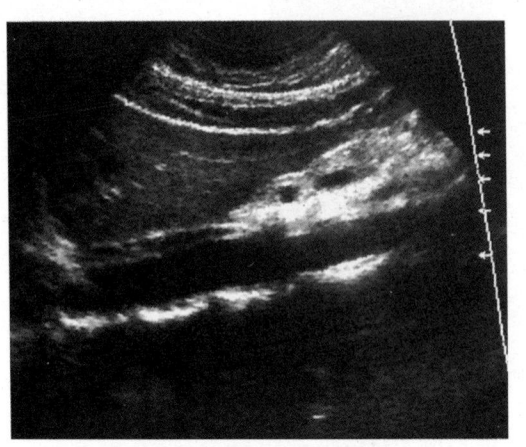

Labeled: **LIVER SAG LT LOBE**

2. Longitudinal image of the left lobe of the liver to include the diaphragm and caudate lobe.

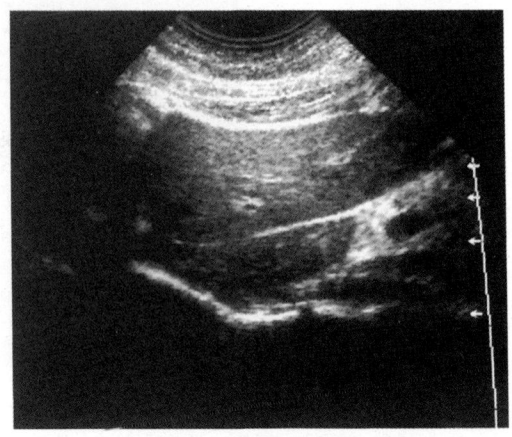

Labeled: **LIVER SAG LT LOBE**

3. Longitudinal image of the right lobe of the liver to include the IVC where it passes through the liver.

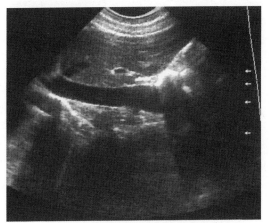

Labeled: **LIVER SAG RT LOBE**

4. Longitudinal image of the right lobe of the liver to include the main lobar fissure, gallbladder, and portal vein.

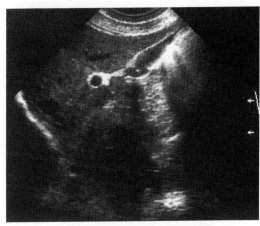

Labeled: **LIVER SAG RT LOBE**

PART III

5. Longitudinal image of the right lobe of the liver to include part of the right kidney for parenchyma comparison.

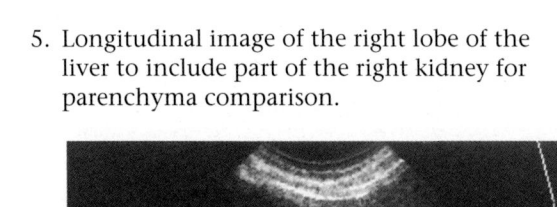

Labeled: **LIVER SAG RT LOBE**

6. Longitudinal image of the right lobe of the liver to include the dome and adjacent pleural space.

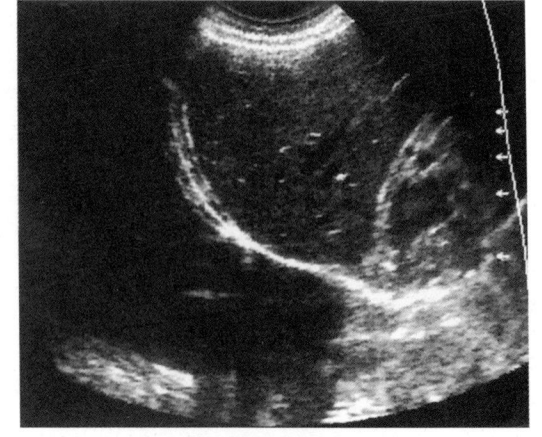

Labeled: **LIVER SAG RT LOBE**

Liver • Axial Images

7. Axial image of the left lobe of the liver to include its lateral margin.

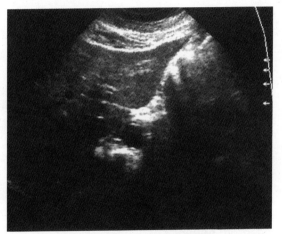

Labeled: **LIVER TRV LT LOBE**

PART III

8. Axial image of the left lobe of the liver to include the ligamentum teres.

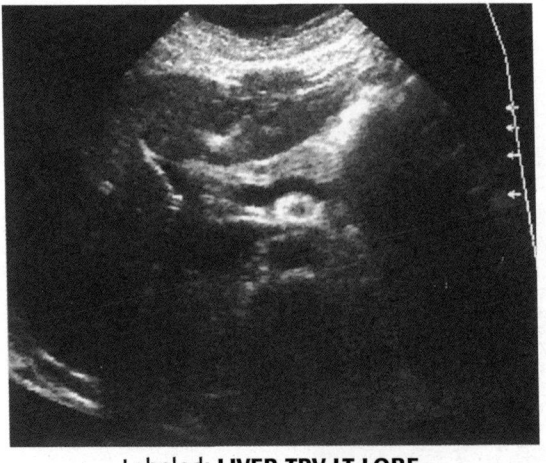

Labeled: **LIVER TRV LT LOBE**

SCANNING TIP: Depending on liver size and shape, it may be possible to document an axial image of the left lobe that includes both the lateral margin and ligamentum teres. If so, label the image as:
LIVER TRV LT LOBE

9. Axial image of the right lobe of the liver to include the hepatic veins.

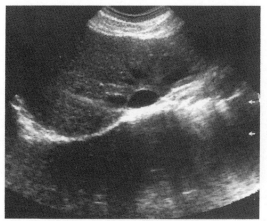

Labeled: **LIVER TRV RT LOBE**

10. Axial image of the right lobe of the liver to include the right and left branches of the portal vein.

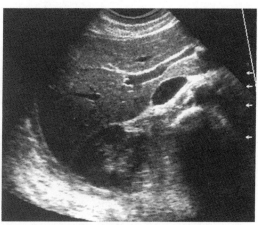

Labeled: **LIVER TRV RT LOBE**

11. Axial image of the right lobe of the liver to include the right lateral inferior lobe.

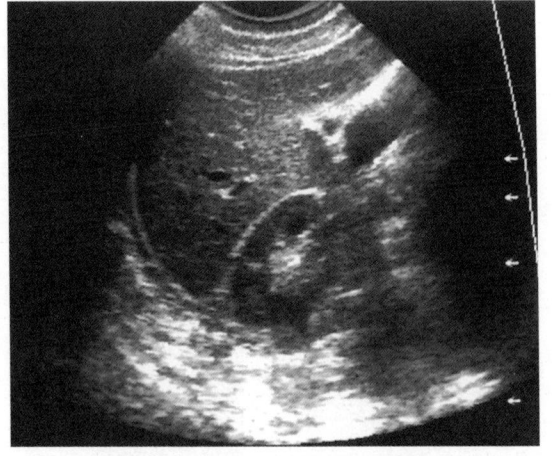

Labeled: **LIVER TRV RT LOBE**

12. Axial image of the right lobe of the liver to include the dome and adjacent pleural space.

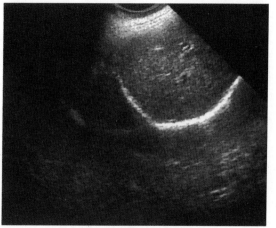

Labeled: **LIVER TRV RT LOBE**

SCANNING TIP: Routine measurements of the liver are not required.

Aorta • Longitudinal Image

SCANNING TIP: The images of the aorta may be included with the liver images if the aorta is well visualized.

13. Longitudinal image of the proximal and middle aorta.

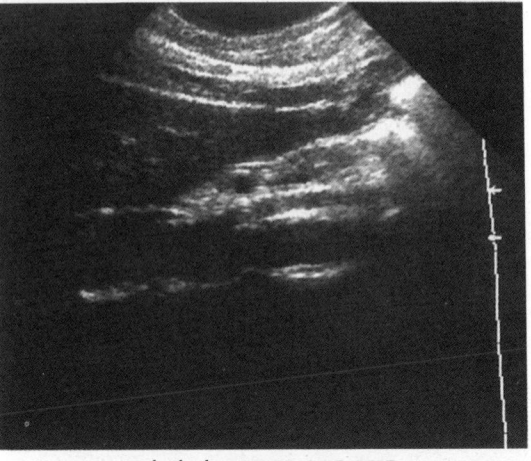

Labeled: **AORTA SAG MID**

Aorta • Axial Image

14. Axial image of the middle aorta at the level of the renal arteries.

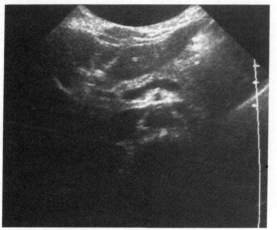

Labeled: **AORTA TRV MID**

Inferior Vena Cava • Longitudinal Image

> **SCANNING TIP:** The images of the IVC may be included with the liver images if the IVC is well visualized.

15. Longitudinal image of the distal and middle IVC.

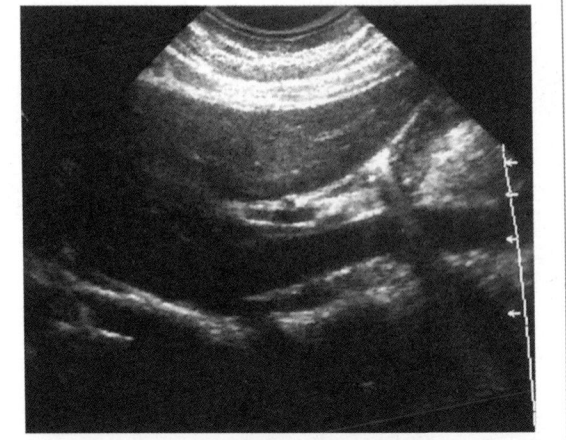

Labeled: **IVC SAG DISTAL**

Inferior Vena Cava • Axial Image

16. Axial image of the distal IVC to include the hepatic veins.

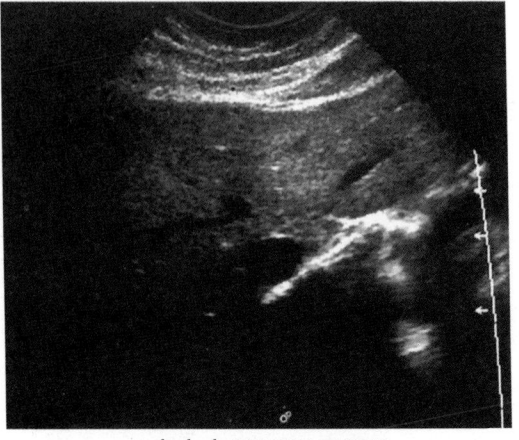

Labeled: **IVC TRV DISTAL**

Gallbladder and Biliary Tract • First Position

SCANNING TIP: When the gallbladder and biliary tract are the areas of interest, they are routinely surveyed in 2 different patient positions and the gallbladder is documented in both positions.

Gallbladder • Longitudinal Images

17. Long axis image of the gallbladder.

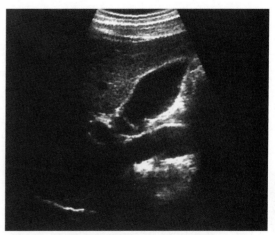

Labeled: **GB SAG LONG AXIS**

PART III

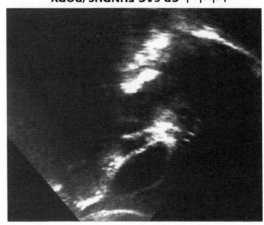

Labeled: GB SAG FUNDUS/BODY

18. Longitudinal image of the gallbladder fundus and body.

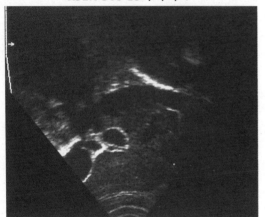

Labeled: GB SAG NECK

19. Longitudinal image of the gallbladder neck.

Gallbladder • Axial Images

20. Axial image of the gallbladder fundus.

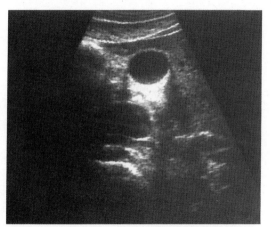

Labeled: **GB TRV FUNDUS**

21. Axial image of the gallbladder body.

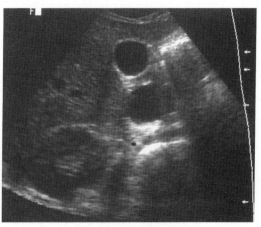

Labeled: **GB TRV BODY**

22. Axial image of the gallbladder neck.

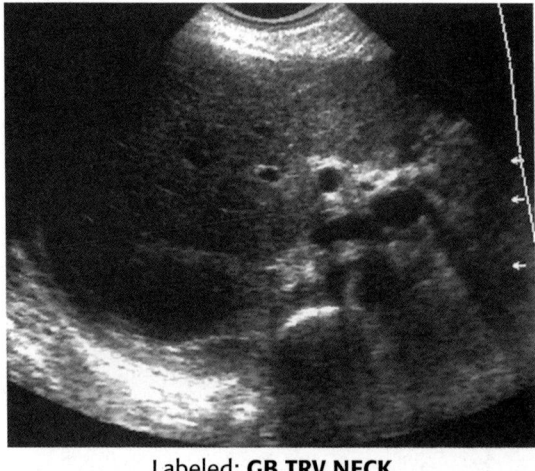

Labeled: **GB TRV NECK**

Biliary Tract • Longitudinal Images

SCANNING TIP: Biliary tract images may be magnified to aid interpretation.

SCANNING TIP: The CHD image may be omitted if the CHD was visualized on the gallbladder long axis image.

SCANNING TIP: Biliary tract images may be taken in the second patient position if they were better visualized there during the survey.

23. Longitudinal image of the CHD.

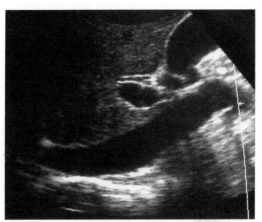

Labeled: **SAG CHD**

24. Longitudinal image of the common bile duct *with anterior to posterior measurement at the widest margins of the lumen.*

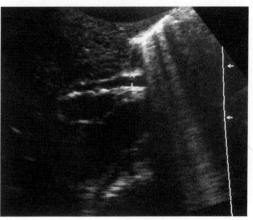

Labeled: **SAG CBD**

25. Same image as number 24 *without measurement calipers*.

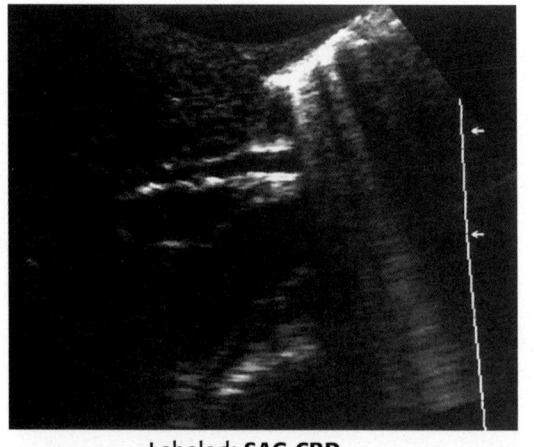

Labeled: **SAG CBD**

Gallbladder and Biliary Tract • Second Position
Gallbladder • Longitudinal Image

26. Long axis image of the gallbladder.

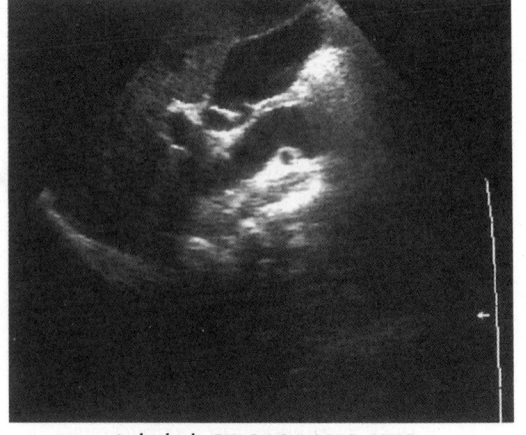

Labeled: **GB SAG LONG AXIS**

Gallbladder • *Axial Image*

27. Axial image of the gallbladder fundus.

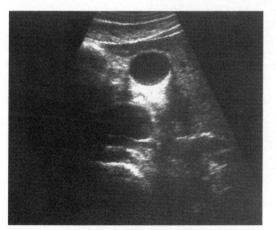

Labeled: **GB TRV FUNDUS**

Pancreas • Longitudinal Images

28. Long axis image of the pancreas to include as much head, uncinate, neck, body, tail, and pancreatic duct as possible.

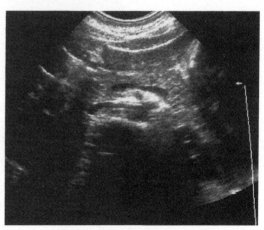

Labeled: **PANC TRV LONG AXIS**

PART III

29. Longitudinal image of the pancreas head, to include the uncinate process and common bile duct (if bile filled).

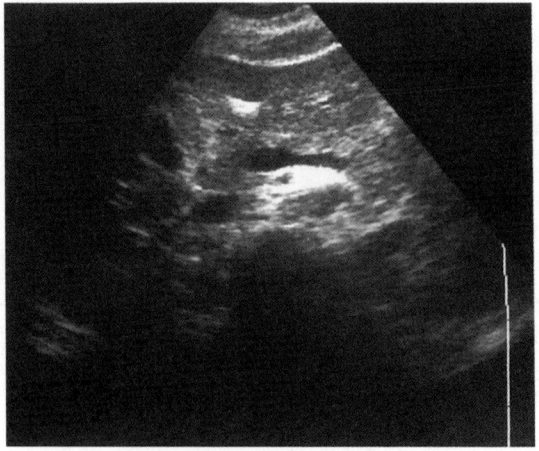

Labeled: **PANC TRV HEAD**

Pancreas • Axial Image

30. Axial image of the pancreas head to include the common bile duct (if bile filled).

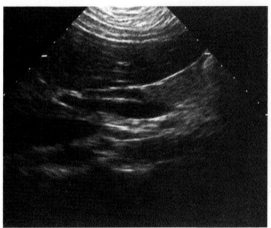

Labeled: **PANC SAG HEAD**

SCANNING TIP: In some cases, a portion or all of the pancreas cannot be visualized because of overlying bowel gas and the patient cannot be given fluids to displace the gas. When this occurs, and every effort has been made to image the pancreas, take the required images in the designated areas and add "AREA" to the labeling.

Right Kidney • Longitudinal Image

31. Long axis image of the right kidney.

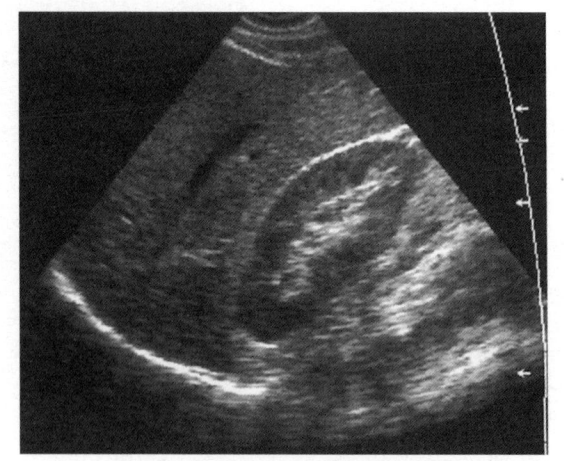

Labeled: **RT KID SAG LONG AXIS**

SCANNING TIP: Take an additional image of the superior and/or inferior poles if they are not clearly represented on the long axis image. Label accordingly.

32. Axial image of the right kidney midportion to include the hilum.

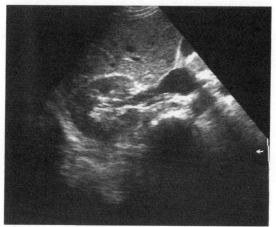

Labeled: **RT KID TRV MID**

Left Kidney • Longitudinal Image

33. Long axis image of the left kidney.

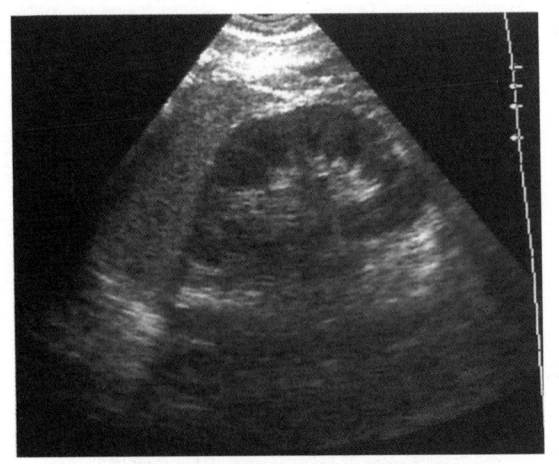

Labeled: **LT KID COR LONG AXIS**

SCANNING TIP: Take an additional image of the superior and/or inferior poles if they are not clearly represented on the long axis image. Label accordingly.

Left Kidney • Axial Image

34. Axial image of the left kidney midportion to include the hilum.

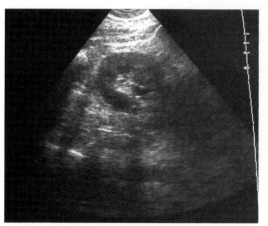

Labeled: **LT KID LT TRV MID**

Spleen • Longitudinal Image

35. Long axis or longitudinal image of the spleen to include the adjacent pleural space superiorly and portion of the left kidney inferiorly.

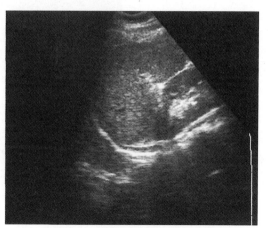

Labeled: **SPLEEN COR LONG AXIS or SPLEEN COR**

Spleen • Axial Image

36. Axial image of the spleen to include the anterior and posterior margins.

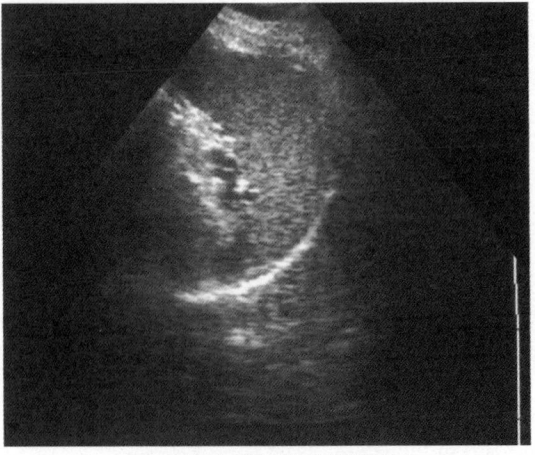

Labeled: **SPLEEN LT TRV**

Pancreas Study With Full Abdomen

Liver • Longitudinal Images

1. Longitudinal image of the left lobe of the liver to include the inferior margin and the aorta.

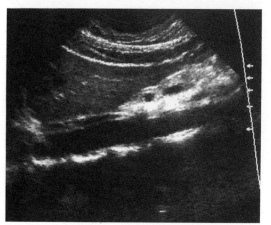

Labeled: **LIVER SAG LT LOBE**

2. Longitudinal image of the left lobe of the liver to include the diaphragm and caudate lobe.

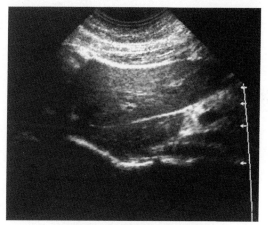

Labeled: **LIVER SAG LT LOBE**

PART III

3. Longitudinal image of the right lobe of the liver to include the IVC where it passes through the liver.

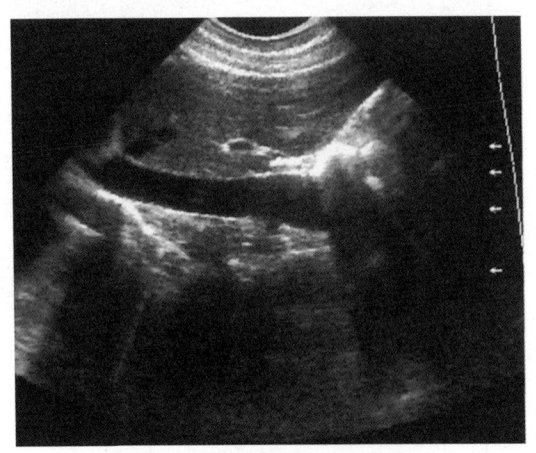

Labeled: **LIVER SAG RT LOBE**

4. Longitudinal image of the right lobe of the liver to include the main lobar fissure, gallbladder, and portal vein.

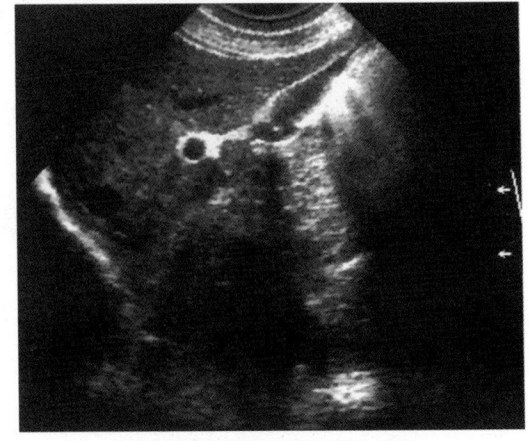

Labeled: **LIVER SAG RT LOBE**

5. Longitudinal image of the right lobe of the liver to include part of the right kidney for parenchyma comparison.

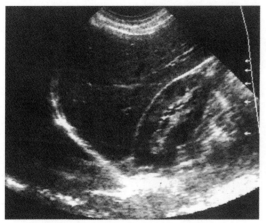

Labeled: **LIVER SAG RT LOBE**

6. Longitudinal image of the right lobe of the liver to include the dome and adjacent pleural space.

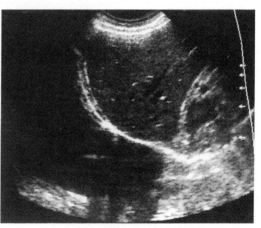

Labeled: **LIVER SAG RT LOBE**

Liver • Axial Images

7. Axial image of the left lobe of the liver to include its lateral margin.

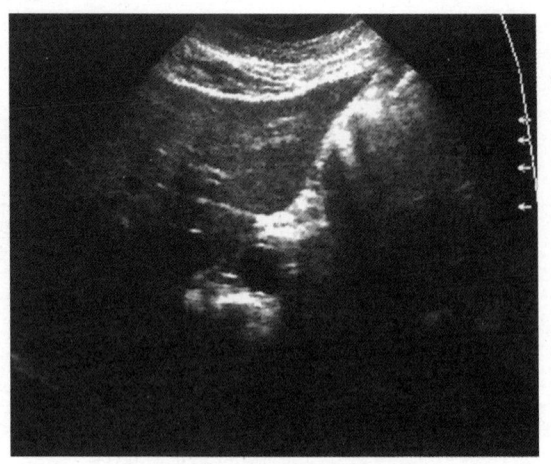

Labeled: **LIVER TRV LT LOBE**

8. Axial image of the left lobe of the liver to include the ligamentum teres.

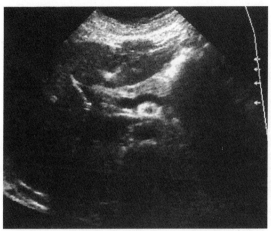

Labeled: **LIVER TRV LT LOBE**

SCANNING TIP: Depending on liver size and shape, it may be possible to document an axial image of the left lobe that includes both the lateral margin and ligamentum teres. If so, label the image as follows:
LIVER TRV LT LOBE

9. Axial image of the right lobe of the liver to include the hepatic veins.

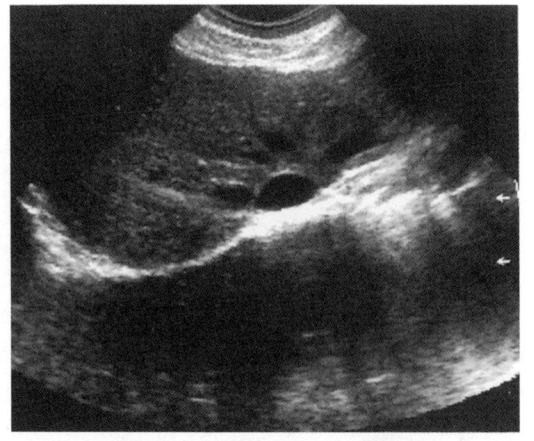

Labeled: **LIVER TRV RT LOBE**

10. Axial image of the right lobe of the liver to include the right and left branches of the portal vein.

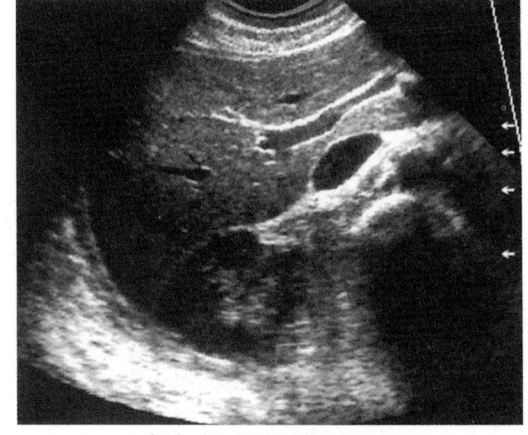

Labeled: **LIVER TRV RT LOBE**

11. Axial image of the right lobe of the liver to include the right lateral inferior lobe.

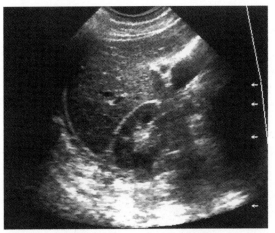

Labeled: **LIVER TRV RT LOBE**

12. Axial image of the right lobe of the liver to include the dome and adjacent pleural space.

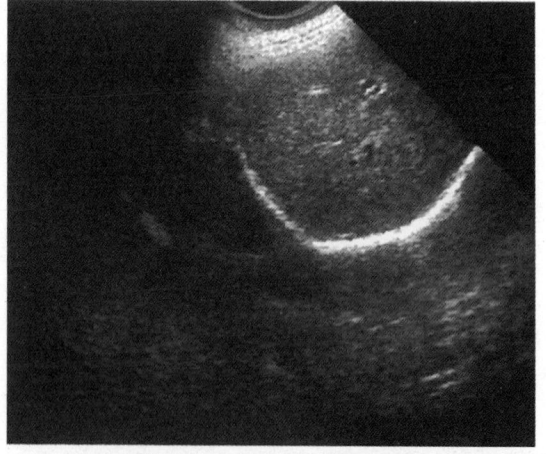

Labeled: **LIVER TRV RT LOBE**

SCANNING TIP: Routine measurements of the liver are not required.

Aorta • Longitudinal Image

> **SCANNING TIP:** The images of the aorta may be included with the liver images if the aorta is well visualized.

13. Longitudinal image of the proximal and middle aorta.

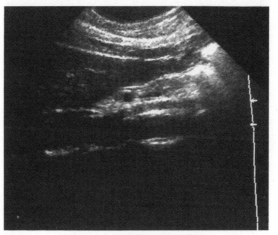

Labeled: **AORTA SAG MID**

PART III

Aorta • Axial Image

14. Axial image of the middle aorta at the level of the renal arteries.

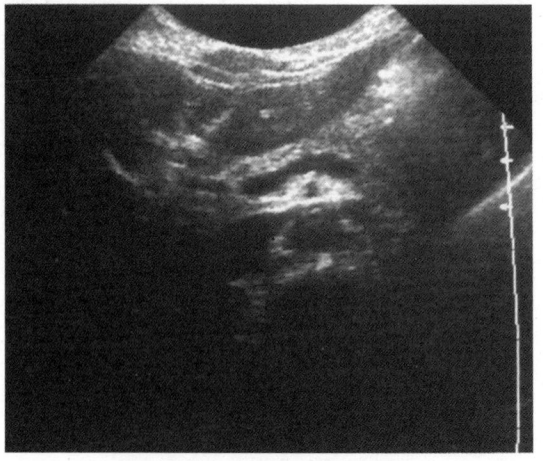

Labeled: **AORTA TRV MID**

Inferior Vena Cava • Longitudinal Image

SCANNING TIP: The images of the IVC may be included with the liver images if the IVC is well visualized.

15. Longitudinal image of the distal and middle IVC.

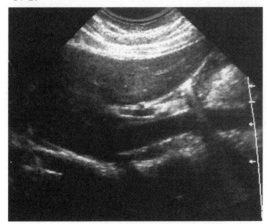

Labeled: **IVC SAG DISTAL**

Inferior Vena Cava • Axial Image

16. Axial image of the distal IVC to include the hepatic veins.

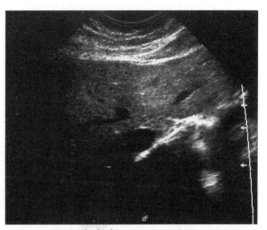

Labeled: **IVC TRV DISTAL**

PART III

Gallbladder • Axial Image

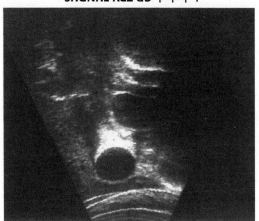

18. Axial image of the gallbladder fundus.

Labeled: **GB TRV FUNDUS**

Gallbladder • Longitudinal Image

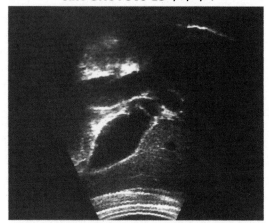

17. Long axis image of the gallbladder.

Labeled: **GB SAG LONG AXIS**

Biliary Tract • Longitudinal Images

SCANNING TIP: Biliary tract images may be magnified to aid interpretation.

SCANNING TIP: The CHD image may be omitted if the CHD was visualized on the gallbladder long axis image.

19. Longitudinal image of the CHD.

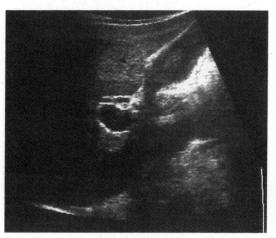

Labeled: **SAG CHD**

PART III

20. Longitudinal image of the common bile duct *with anterior to posterior measurement at the widest margins of the lumen.*

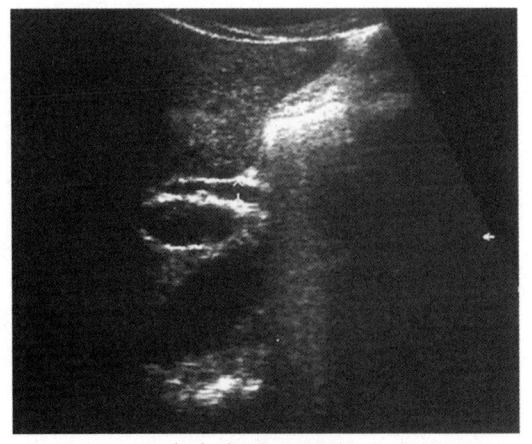

Labeled: **SAG CBD**

21. Same image as number 20 *without measurement calipers.*

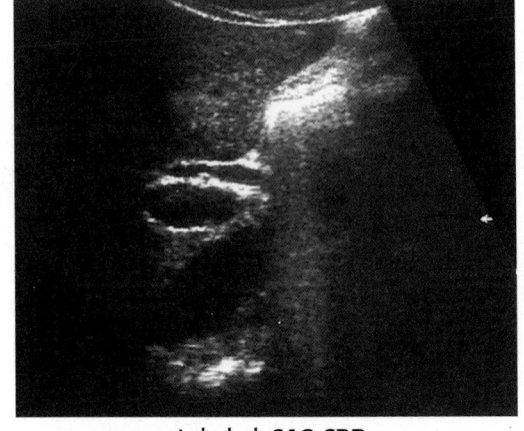

Labeled: **SAG CBD**

Pancreas • Longitudinal Images

22. Long axis image of the pancreas to include as much head, uncinate, neck, body, tail, and pancreatic duct as possible.

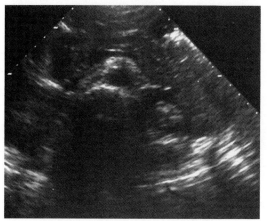

Labeled: **PANC TRV LONG AXIS**

23. Longitudinal image of the pancreas body and neck to include the splenic vein.

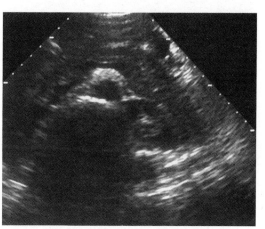

Labeled: **PANC TRV BODY/NECK**

PART III

24. Longitudinal image of the pancreas tail.

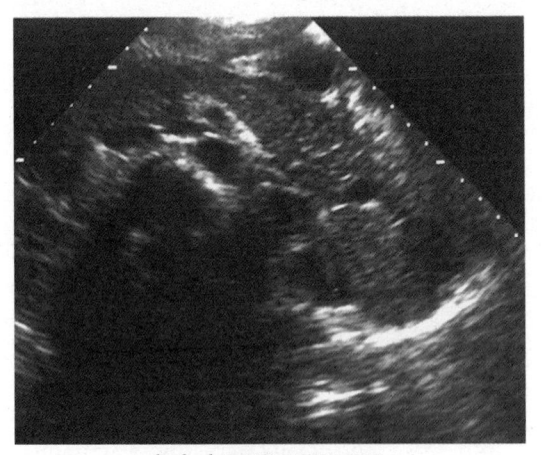

Labeled: **PANC TRV TAIL**

25. Longitudinal image of the pancreas head to include the uncinate process and common bile duct (if bile filled).

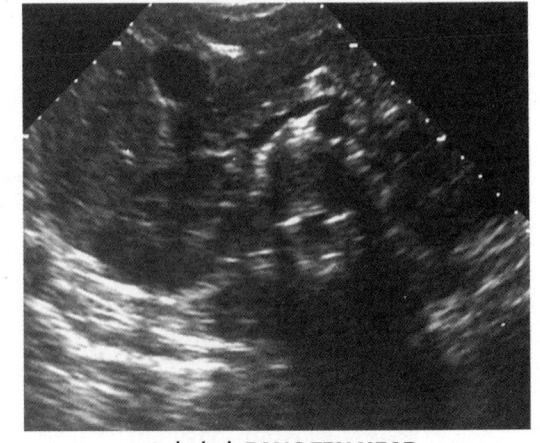

Labeled: **PANC TRV HEAD**

Pancreas • Axial Images

26. Axial image of the pancreas head to include the common bile duct (if bile filled).

27. Axial image of the pancreas neck and uncinate process to include the superior mesenteric vein.

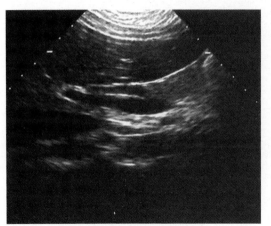

Labeled: **PANC SAG HEAD**

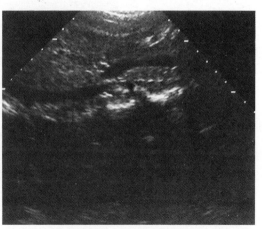

Labeled: **PANC SAG NECK/UNCINATE**

PART III

28. Axial image of the pancreas body to include the splenic vein.

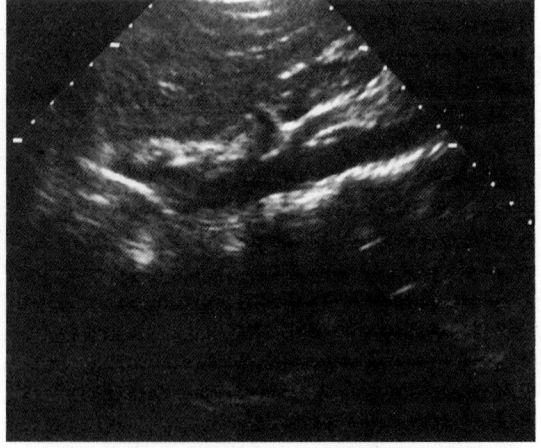

Labeled: **PANC SAG BODY**

29. Axial image of the pancreas tail.

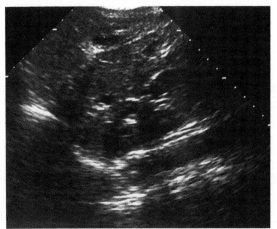

Labeled: **PANC SAG TAIL**

SCANNING TIP: In some cases, a portion or all of the pancreas cannot be visualized because of overlying bowel gas and the patient cannot be given fluids to displace the gas. When this occurs, and every effort has been made to image the pancreas, take the required images in the designated areas and add "AREA" to the labeling.

PART III

Right Kidney • Longitudinal Image

30. Long axis image of the right kidney.

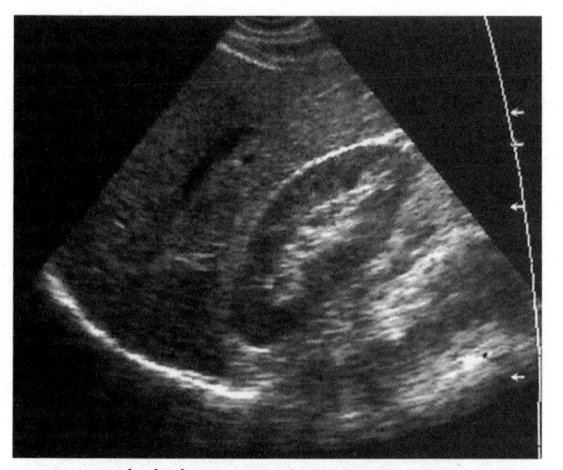

Labeled: **RT KID SAG LONG AXIS**

SCANNING TIP: Take an additional image of the superior and/or inferior poles if they are not clearly represented on the long axis image. Label accordingly.

Right Kidney • Axial Image

31. Axial image of the right kidney midportion to include the hilum.

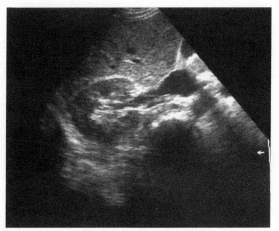

Labeled: **RT KID TRV MID**

Left Kidney • Longitudinal Image

32. Long axis image of the left kidney.

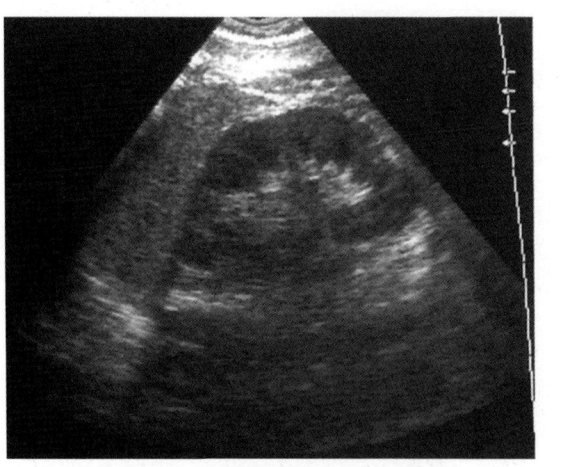

Labeled: **LT KID COR LONG AXIS**

SCANNING TIP: Take an additional image of the superior and/or inferior poles if they are not clearly represented on the long axis image. Label accordingly.

Left Kidney • Axial Image

33. Axial image of the left kidney midportion to include the hilum.

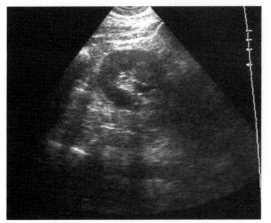

Labeled: **LT KID LT TRV MID**

Spleen • Longitudinal Image

34. Long axis or longitudinal image of the spleen to include the adjacent pleural space superiorly and portion of the left kidney inferiorly.

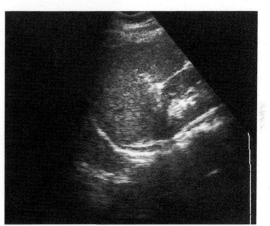

Labeled: **SPLEEN COR LONG AXIS or SPLEEN COR**

PART III

Spleen • Axial Image

35. Axial image of the spleen to include the anterior and posterior margins.

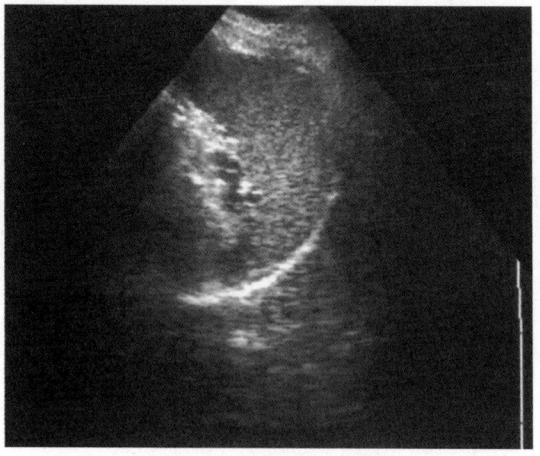

Labeled: **SPLEEN LT TRV**

Renal Study With Full Abdomen

Liver • Longitudinal Images

1. Longitudinal image of the left lobe of the liver to include the inferior margin and the aorta.

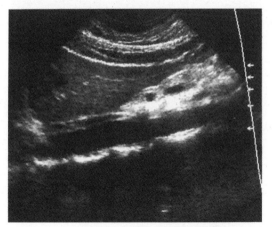

Labeled: **LIVER SAG LT LOBE**

2. Longitudinal image of the left lobe of the liver to include the diaphragm and caudate lobe.

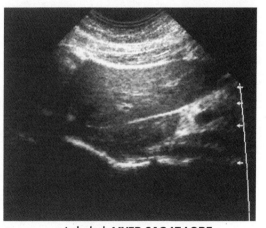

Labeled: **LIVER SAG LT LOBE**

PART III

3. Longitudinal image of the right lobe of the liver to include the IVC where it passes through the liver.

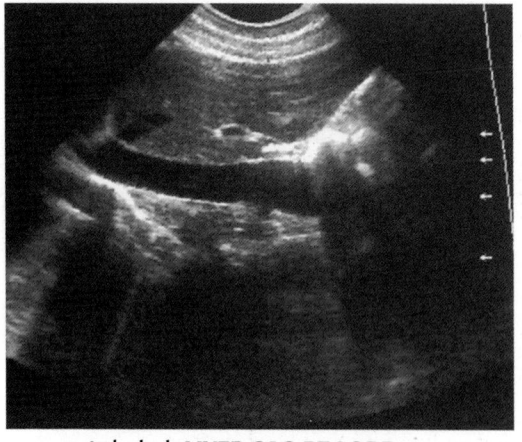

Labeled: **LIVER SAG RT LOBE**

4. Longitudinal image of the right lobe of the liver to include the main lobar fissure, gallbladder, and portal vein.

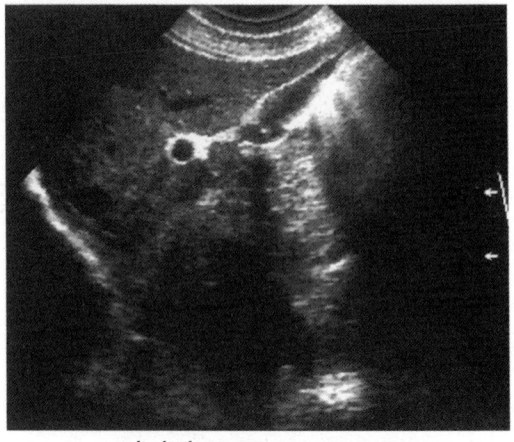

Labeled: **LIVER SAG RT LOBE**

5. Longitudinal image of the right lobe of the liver to include part of the right kidney for parenchyma comparison.

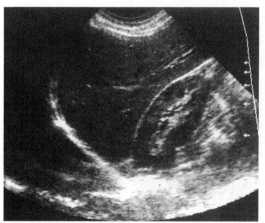

Labeled: **LIVER SAG RT LOBE**

6. Longitudinal image of the right lobe of the liver to include the dome and adjacent pleural space.

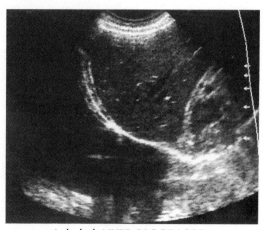

Labeled: **LIVER SAG RT LOBE**

Liver • Axial Images

7. Axial image of the left lobe of the liver to include its lateral margin.

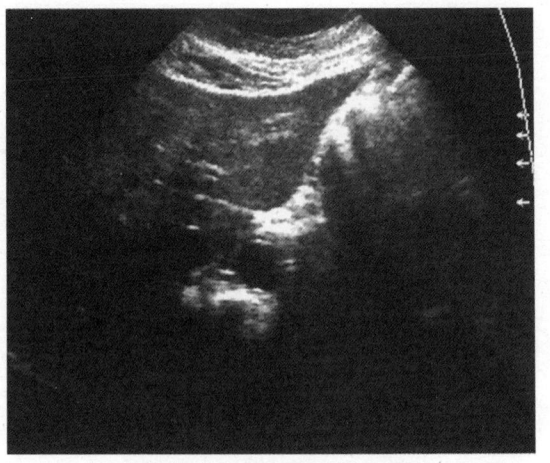

Labeled: **LIVER TRV LT LOBE**

8. Axial image of the left lobe of the liver to include the ligamentum teres.

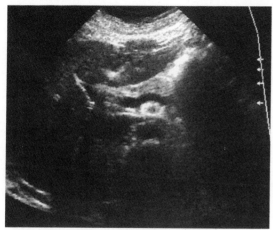

Labeled: **LIVER TRV LT LOBE**

SCANNING TIP: Depending on liver size and shape, it may be possible to document an axial image of the left lobe that includes both the lateral margin and ligamentum teres. If so, label the image as follows:
LIVER TRV LT LOBE

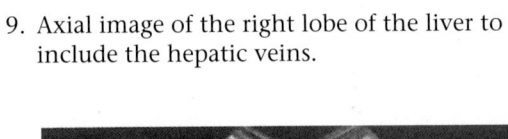

9. Axial image of the right lobe of the liver to include the hepatic veins.

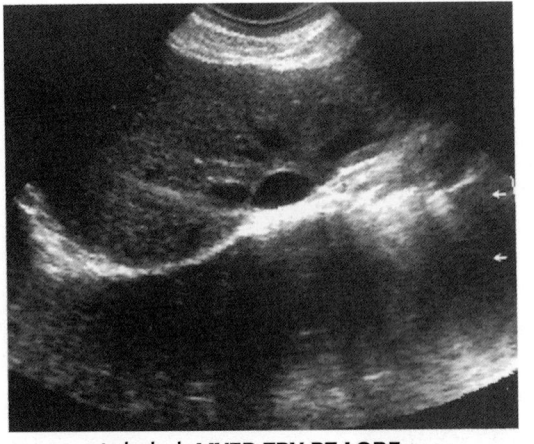

Labeled: **LIVER TRV RT LOBE**

10. Axial image of the right lobe of the liver to include the right and left branches of the portal vein.

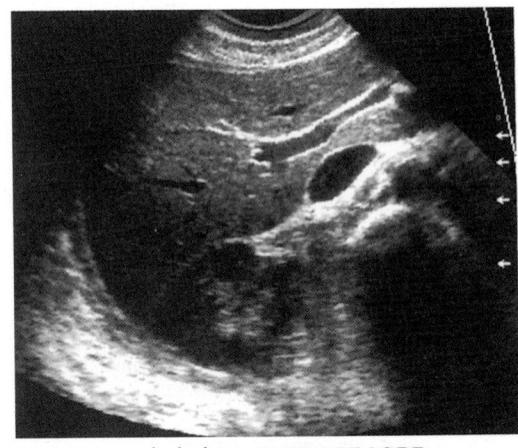

Labeled: **LIVER TRV RT LOBE**

11. Axial image of the right lobe of the liver to include the right lateral inferior lobe.

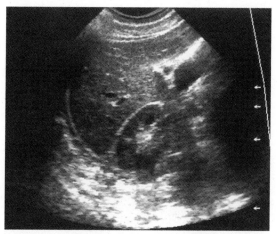

Labeled: **LIVER TRV RT LOBE**

12. Axial image of the right lobe of the liver to include the dome and adjacent pleural space.

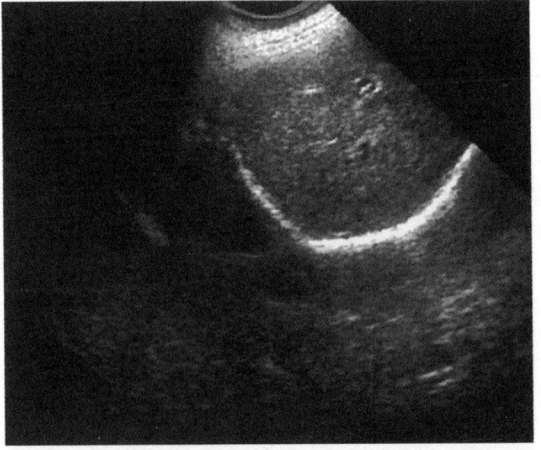

Labeled: **LIVER TRV RT LOBE**

SCANNING TIP: Routine measurements of the liver are not required.

Aorta • Longitudinal Image

> **SCANNING TIP:** The images of the aorta may be included with the liver images if the aorta is well visualized.

13. Longitudinal image of the proximal and middle aorta.

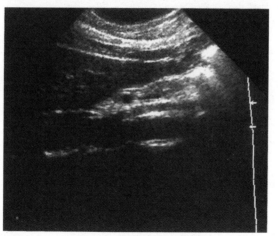

Labeled: **AORTA SAG MID**

Aorta • Axial Image

14. Axial image of the middle aorta at the level of the renal arteries.

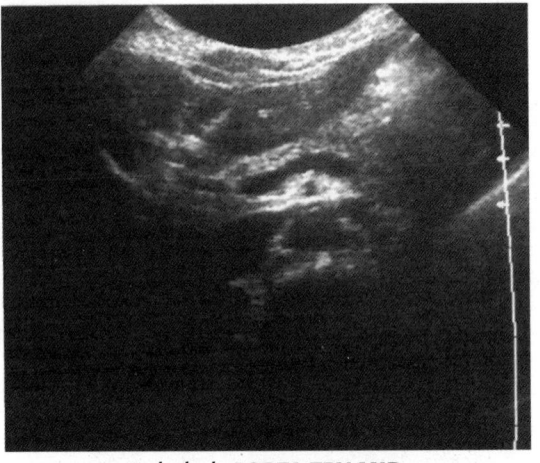

Labeled: **AORTA TRV MID**

Inferior Vena Cava • Longitudinal Images

> **SCANNING TIP:** The images of the IVC may be included with the liver images if the IVC is well visualized.

15. Longitudinal image of the distal and middle IVC.

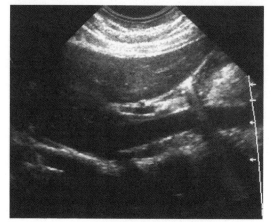

Labeled: **IVC SAG DISTAL**

Inferior Vena Cava • Axial Images

16. Axial image of the distal IVC to include the hepatic veins.

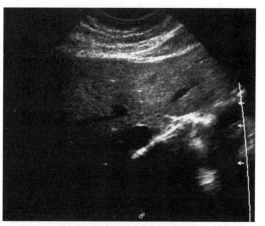

Labeled: **IVC TRV DISTAL**

Gallbladder • Longitudinal Image

17. Long axis image of the gallbladder.

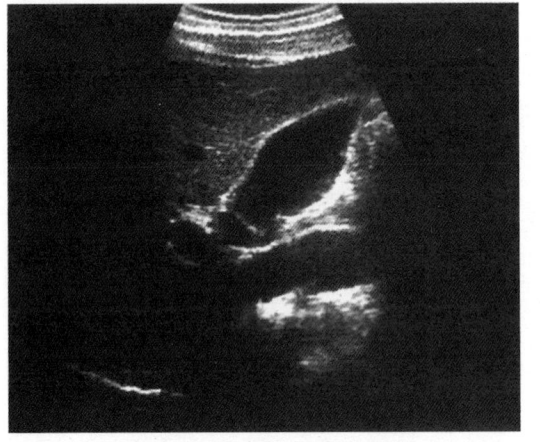

Labeled: **GB SAG LONG AXIS**

Gallbladder • Axial Image

18. Axial image of the gallbladder fundus.

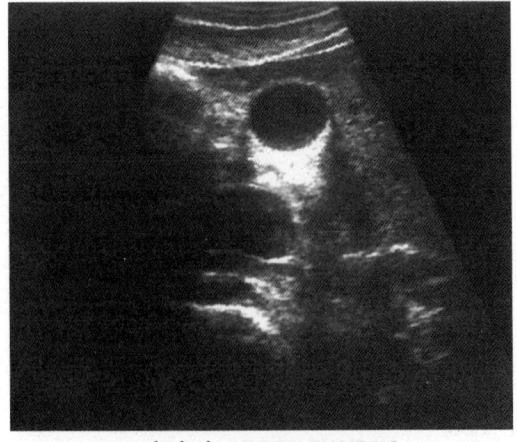

Labeled: **GB TRV FUNDUS**

Biliary Tract • Longitudinal Images

> **SCANNING TIP:** Biliary tract images may be magnified to aid interpretation.
>
> **SCANNING TIP:** The CHD image may be omitted if the CHD was visualized on the gallbladder long axis image.

19. Longitudinal image of the CHD.

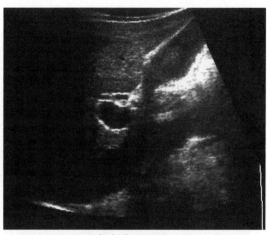

Labeled: **SAG CHD**

PART III

20. Longitudinal image of the common bile duct *with anterior to posterior measurement at the widest margins of the lumen.*

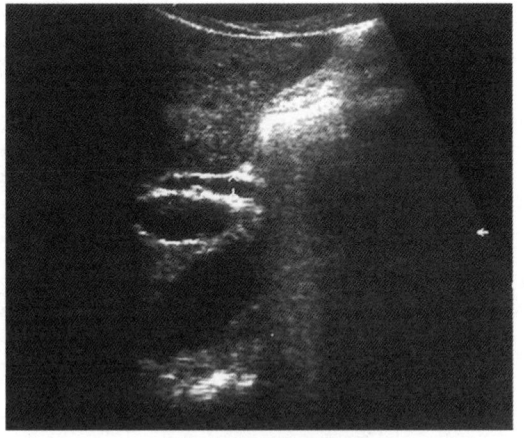

Labeled: **SAG CBD**

21. Same image as number 20 *without measurement calipers.*

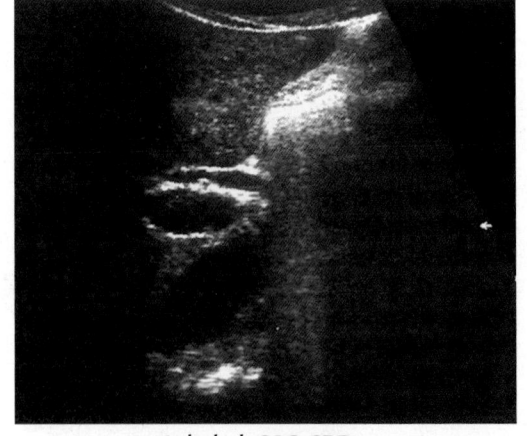

Labeled: **SAG CBD**

Pancreas • Longitudinal Images

22. Long axis image of the pancreas to include as much head, uncinate, neck, body, tail, and pancreatic duct as possible.

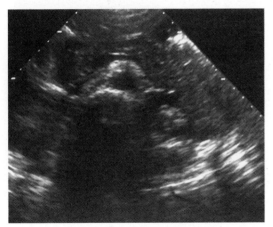

Labeled: **PANC TRV LONG AXIS**

23. Longitudinal image of the pancreas head, to include the uncinate process and common bile duct (if bile filled).

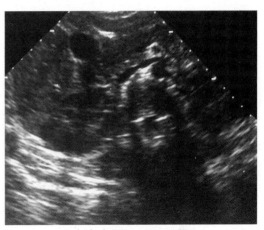

Labeled: **PANC TRV HEAD**

PART III

Pancreas • Axial Image

24. Axial image of the pancreas head to include the common bile duct (if bile filled).

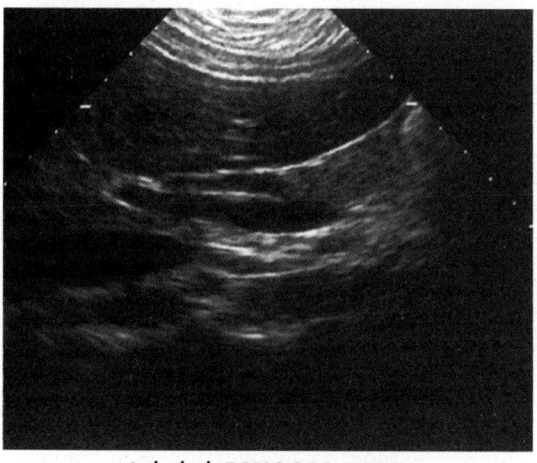

SCANNING TIP: In some cases, a portion or all of the pancreas cannot be visualized because of overlying bowel gas and the patient cannot be given fluids to displace the gas. When this occurs, and every effort has been made to image the pancreas, take the required images in the designated areas and add "AREA" to the labeling.

Labeled: **PANC SAG HEAD**

Right Kidney • Longitudinal Images

25. Long axis image of the right kidney *with superior to inferior measurement.*

26. Same image as number 25, *without measurement calipers.*

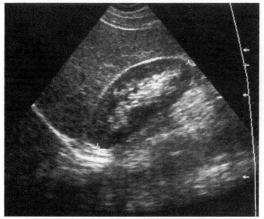

Labeled: **RT KID SAG LONG AXIS**

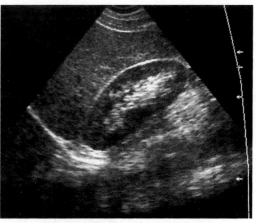

Labeled: **RT KID SAG LONG AXIS**

27. Long axis image of the right kidney *with superior to inferior measurement.*

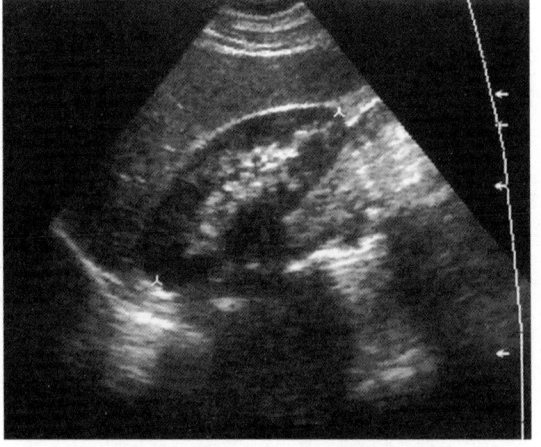

Labeled: **RT KID SAG LONG AXIS**

28. Same image as number 27, *without measurement calipers.*

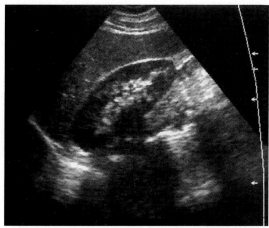

Labeled: **RT KID SAG LONG AXIS**

SCANNING TIP: If the superior and inferior poles were adequately demonstrated on the long axis images, numbers 29 and/or 30 may be omitted.

29. Longitudinal image of the right kidney superior pole.

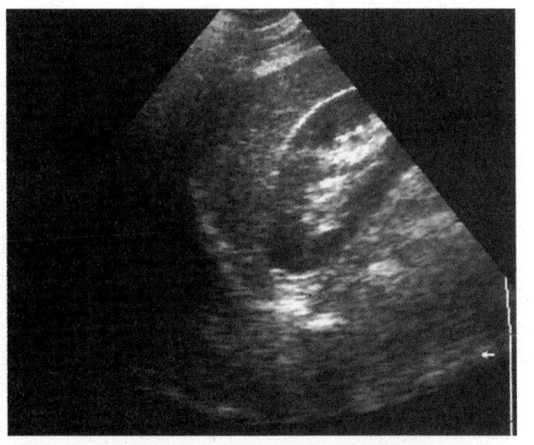

Labeled: **RT KID SAG SUP POLE**

30. Longitudinal image of the right kidney inferior pole.

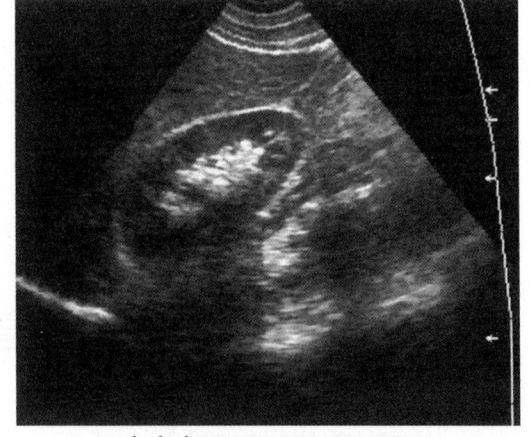

Labeled: **RT KID SAG INF POLE**

31. Longitudinal image of the right kidney just medial to the long axis.

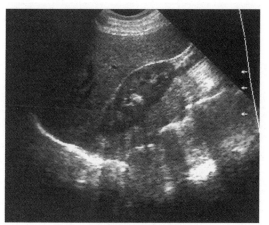

Labeled: **RT KID SAG MED**

32. Longitudinal image of the right kidney just lateral to the long axis to include part of the liver for parenchyma comparison.

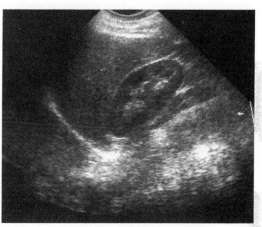

Labeled: **RT KID SAG LAT**

PART III

Right Kidney • Axial Images

33. Axial image of the right kidney superior pole.

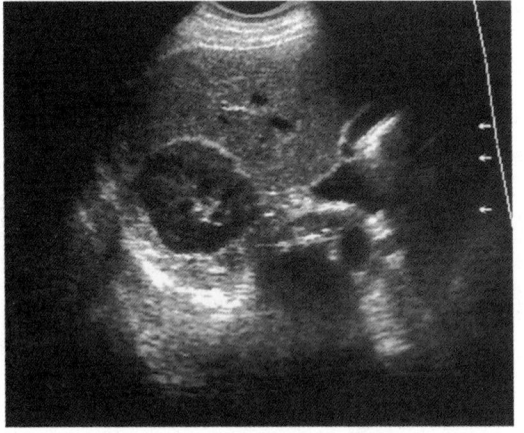

Labeled: **RT KID TRV SUP POLE**

34. Axial image of the right kidney midportion to include the hilum and *anterior to posterior measurement.*

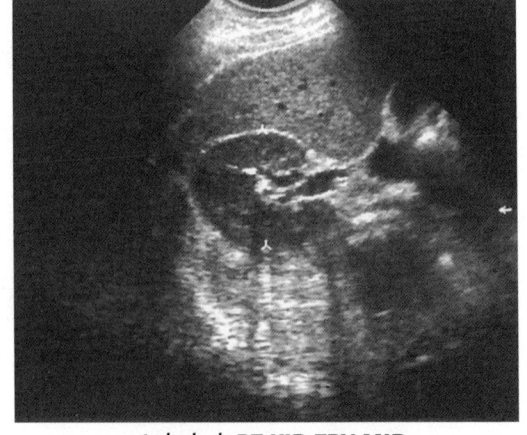

Labeled: **RT KID TRV MID**

35. Same image as number 34, *without measurement calipers.*

36. Axial image of the right kidney inferior pole.

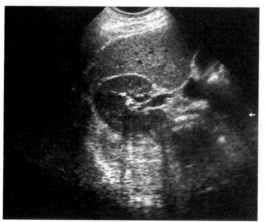

Labeled: **RT KID TRV MID**

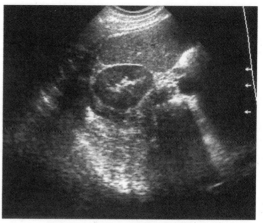

Labeled: **RT KID TRV INF POLE**

Left Kidney • Longitudinal Images

37. Long axis image of the left kidney *with superior to inferior measurement.*

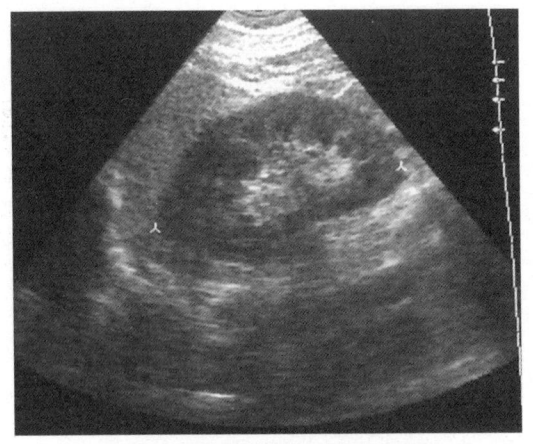

Labeled: **LT KID COR LONG AXIS**

38. Same image as number 37, *without measurement calipers.*

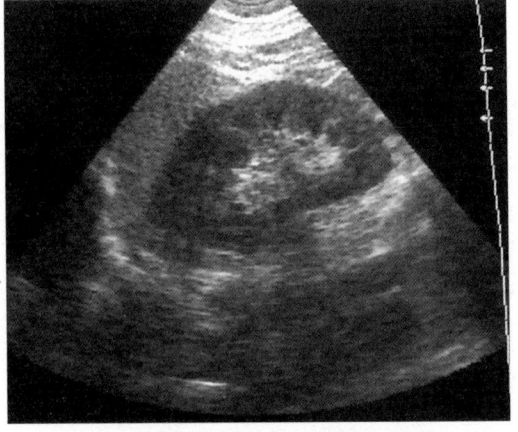

Labeled: **LT KID COR LONG AXIS**

39. Long axis image of the left kidney *with superior to inferior measurement.*

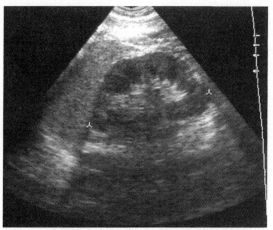

Labeled: **LT KID COR LONG AXIS**

PART III

40. Same image as number 39, *without measurement calipers.*

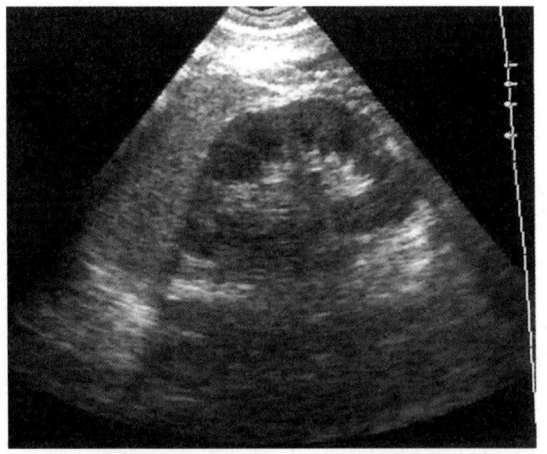

Labeled: **LT KID COR LONG AXIS**

SCANNING TIP: If the superior and inferior poles were adequately demonstrated on the long axis images, numbers 41 and/or 42 may be omitted.

41. Longitudinal image of the left kidney superior pole with part of the spleen for parenchyma comparison.

42. Longitudinal image of the left kidney inferior pole.

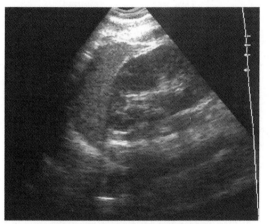

Labeled: **LT KID COR SUP POLE**

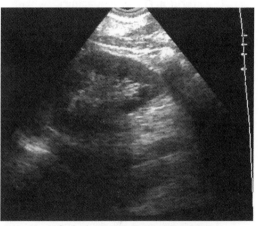

Labeled: **LT KID COR INF POLE**

43. Longitudinal image of the left kidney just anterior to the long axis.

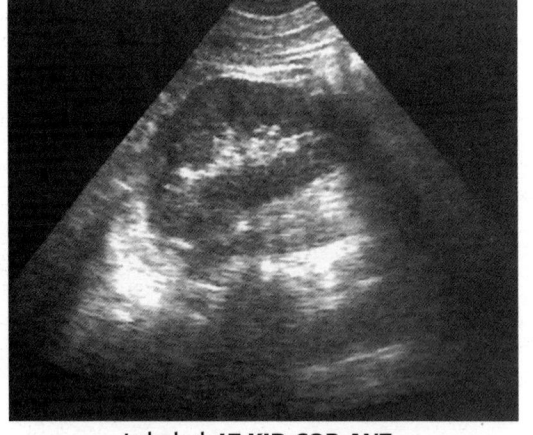

Labeled: **LT KID COR ANT**

44. Longitudinal image of the left kidney just posterior to the long axis.

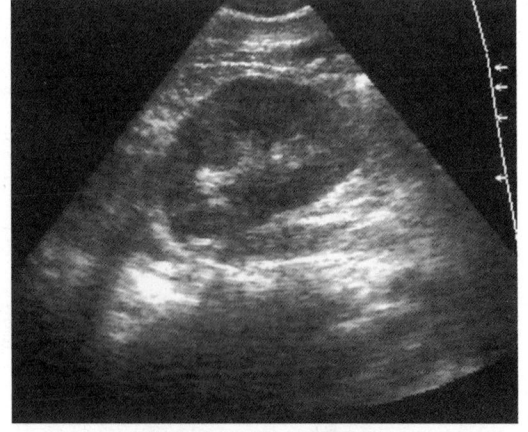

Labeled: **LT KID COR POST**

Left Kidney • Axial Images

45. Axial image of the left kidney superior pole.

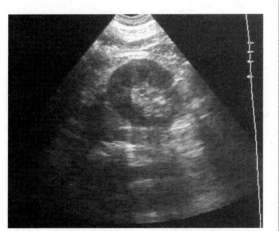

Labeled: **LT KID LT TRV SUP POLE**

46. Axial image of the left kidney midportion to include the hilum and *anterior to posterior measurement.*

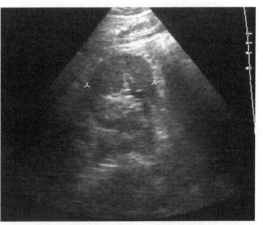

Labeled: **LT KID LT TRV MID**

PART III

47. Same image as number 46, *without measurement calipers*.

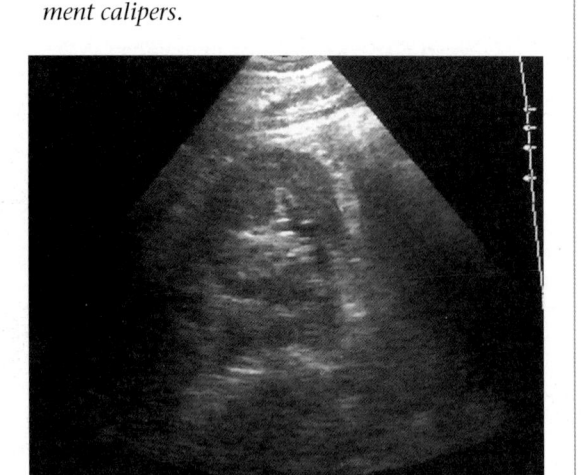

Labeled: **RT KID TRV MID**

48. Axial image of the left kidney inferior pole.

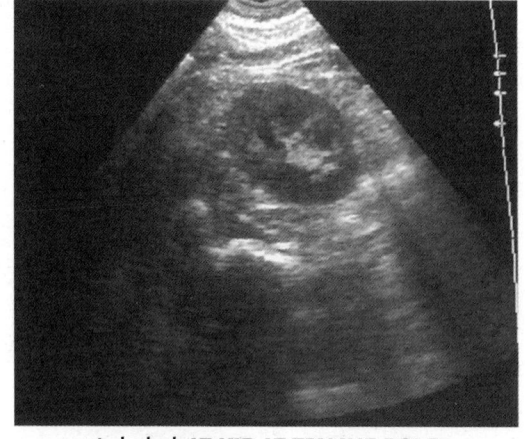

Labeled: **LT KID LT TRV INF POLE**

Spleen • Longitudinal Image

49. Long axis or longitudinal image of the spleen to include the adjacent pleural space superiorly and portion of the left kidney inferiorly.

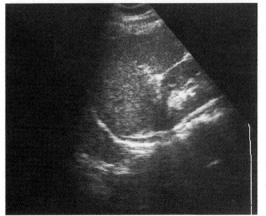

Labeled: **SPLEEN COR LONG AXIS or SPLEEN COR**

Spleen • Axial Image

50. Axial image of the spleen to include the anterior and posterior margins.

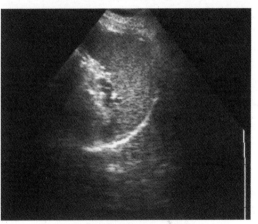

Labeled: **SPLEEN LT TRV**

PART III

Spleen Study With Full Abdomen

Liver • Longitudinal Images

1. Longitudinal image of the left lobe of the liver to include the inferior margin and the aorta.

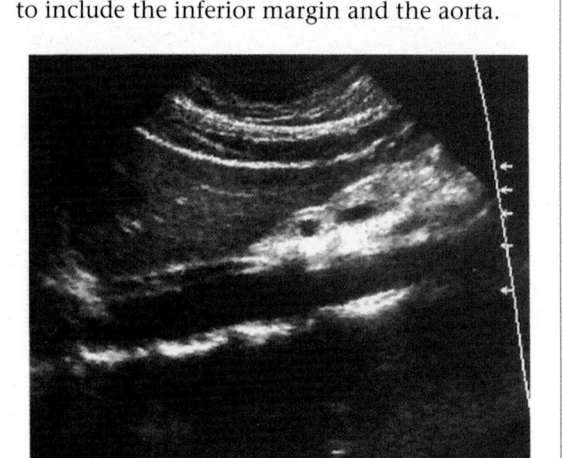

Labeled: **LIVER SAG LT LOBE**

2. Longitudinal image of the left lobe of the liver to include the diaphragm and caudate lobe.

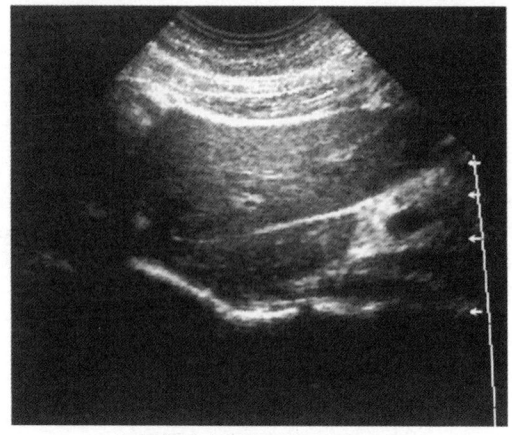

Labeled: **LIVER SAG LT LOBE**

3. Longitudinal image of the right lobe of the liver to include the IVC where it passes through the liver.

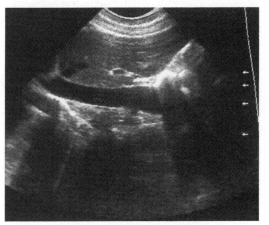

Labeled: **LIVER SAG RT LOBE**

4. Longitudinal image of the right lobe of the liver to include the main lobar fissure, gallbladder, and portal vein.

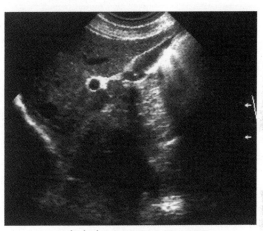

Labeled: **LIVER SAG RT LOBE**

5. Longitudinal image of the right lobe of the liver to include part of the right kidney for parenchyma comparison.

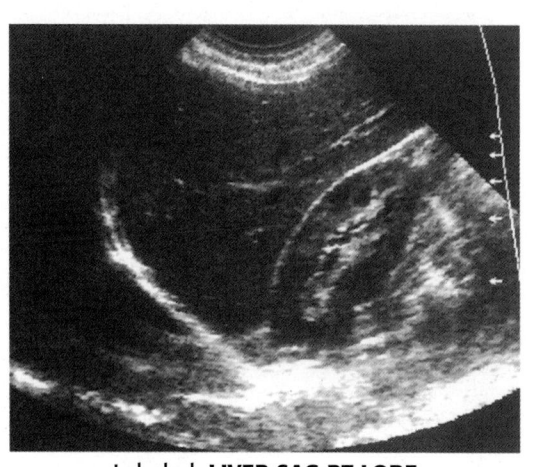

Labeled: **LIVER SAG RT LOBE**

6. Longitudinal image of the right lobe of the liver to include the dome and adjacent pleural space.

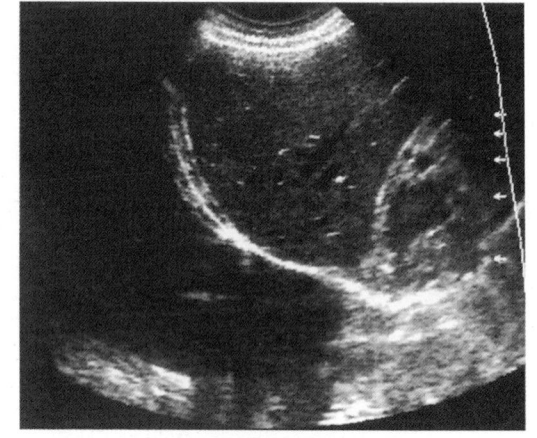

Labeled: **LIVER SAG RT LOBE**

Liver • Axial Images

7. Axial image of the left lobe of the liver to include its lateral margin.

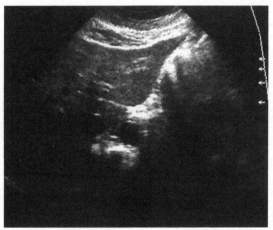

Labeled: **LIVER TRV LT LOBE**

8. Axial image of the left lobe of the liver to include the ligamentum teres.

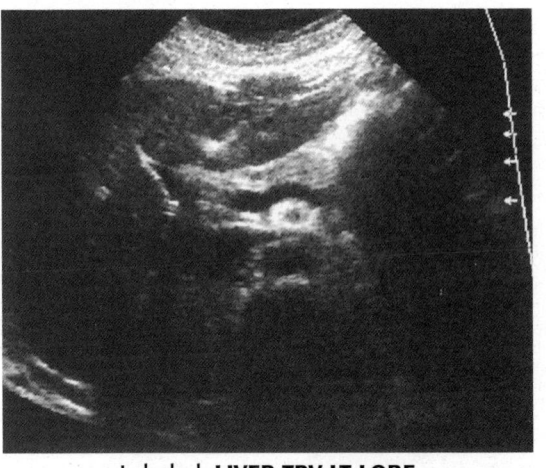

Labeled: **LIVER TRV LT LOBE**

SCANNING TIP: Depending on liver size and shape, it may be possible to document an axial image of the left lobe that includes both the lateral margin and ligamentum teres. If so, label the image as follows:
LIVER TRV LT LOBE

9. Axial image of the right lobe of the liver to include the hepatic veins.

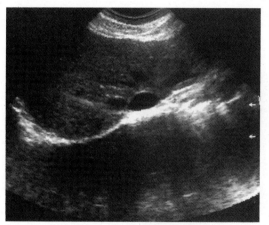

Labeled: **LIVER TRV RT LOBE**

10. Axial image of the right lobe of the liver to include the right and left branches of the portal vein.

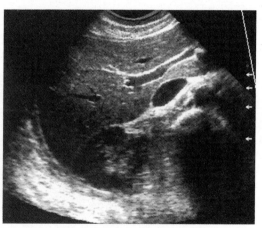

Labeled: **LIVER TRV RT LOBE**

PART III

11. Axial image of the right lobe of the liver to include the right lateral inferior lobe.

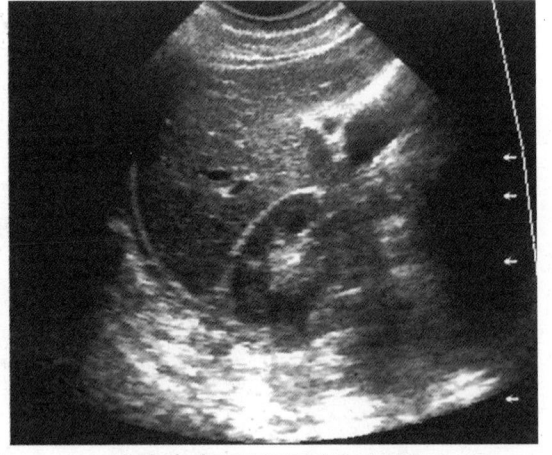

Labeled: **LIVER TRV RT LOBE**

12. Axial image of the right lobe of the liver to include the dome and adjacent pleural space.

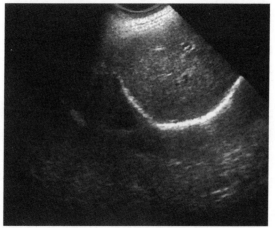

Labeled: **LIVER TRV RT LOBE**

SCANNING TIP: Routine measurements of the liver are not required.

Aorta • Longitudinal Image

SCANNING TIP: The images of the aorta may be included with the liver images if the aorta is well visualized.

13. Longitudinal image of the proximal and middle aorta.

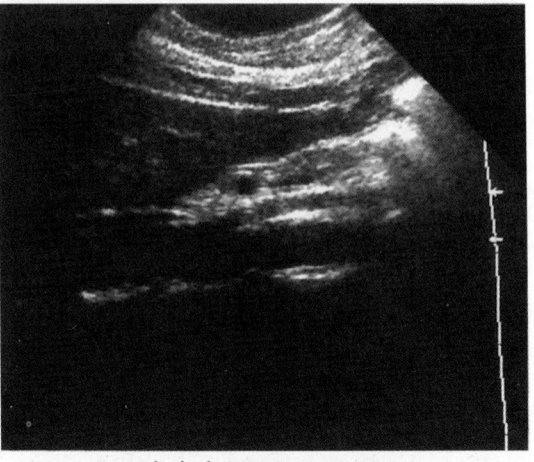

Labeled: **AORTA SAG MID**

Aorta • Axial Image

14. Axial image of the middle aorta at the level of the renal arteries.

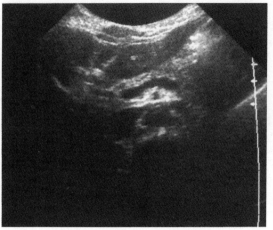

Labeled: **AORTA TRV MID**

Inferior Vena Cava • Longitudinal Image

> **SCANNING TIP:** The images of the IVC may be included with the liver images if the IVC is well visualized.

15. Longitudinal image of the distal and middle IVC.

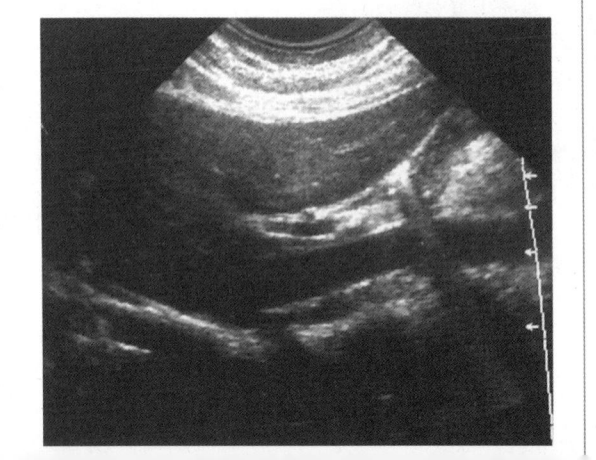

Inferior Vena Cava • Axial Image

16. Axial image of the distal IVC to include the hepatic veins.

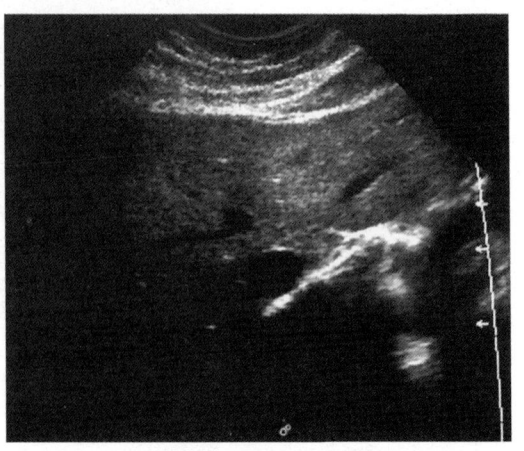

Labeled: **IVC TRV DISTAL**

Gallbladder • Longitudinal Image

17. Long axis image of the gallbladder.

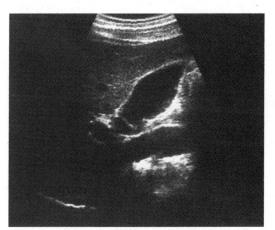

Labeled: **GB SAG LONG AXIS**

Gallbladder • Axial Image

18. Axial image of the gallbladder fundus.

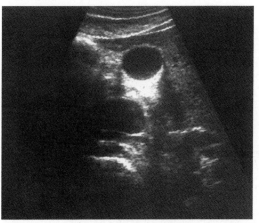

Labeled: **GB TRV FUNDUS**

PART III

Biliary Tract • Longitudinal Images

> **SCANNING TIP:** Biliary tract images may be magnified to aid interpretation.
>
> **SCANNING TIP:** The CHD image may be omitted if the CHD was visualized on the gallbladder long axis image.

19. Longitudinal image of the CHD.

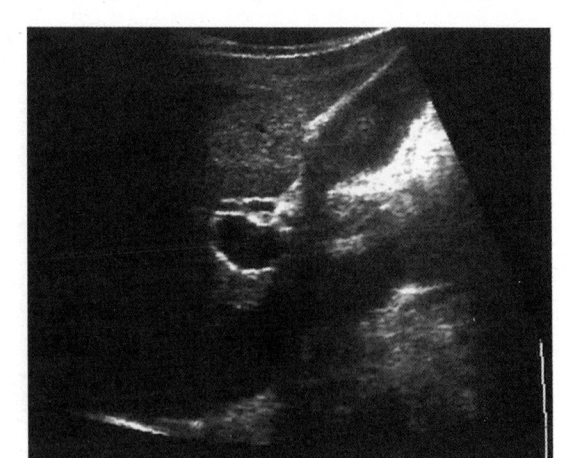

Labeled: **SAG CHD**

20. Longitudinal image of the common bile duct *with anterior to posterior measurement at the widest margins of the lumen.*

21. Same image as number 20 *without measurement calipers.*

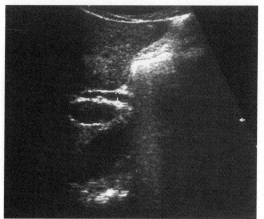

Labeled: **SAG CBD**

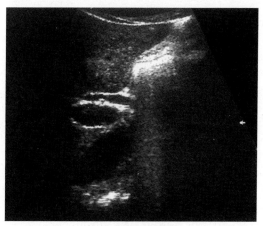

Labeled: **SAG CBD**

PART III

Pancreas • Longitudinal Images

22. Long axis image of the pancreas to include as much head, uncinate, neck, body, tail, and pancreatic duct as possible.

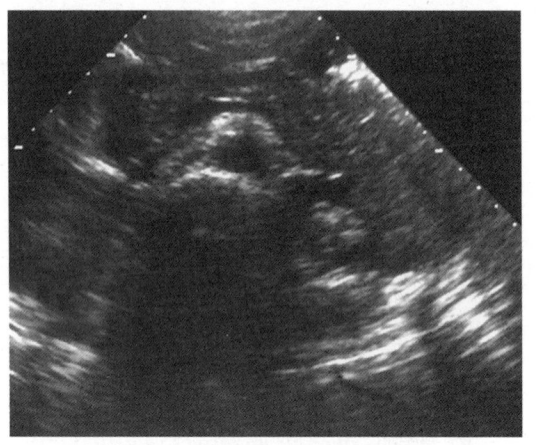

Labeled: **PANC TRV LONG AXIS**

23. Longitudinal image of the pancreas head to include the uncinate process and common bile duct (if bile filled).

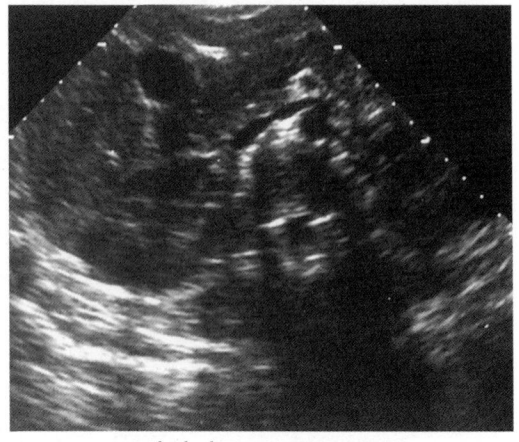

Labeled: **PANC TRV HEAD**

Pancreas • Axial Image

24. Axial image of the pancreas head to include the common bile duct (if bile filled).

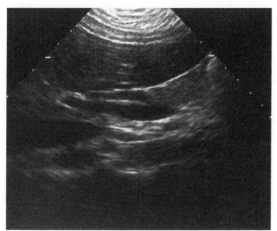

Labeled: **PANC SAG HEAD**

SCANNING TIP: In some cases, a portion or all of the pancreas cannot be visualized because of overlying bowel gas and the patient cannot be given fluids to displace the gas. When this occurs, and every effort has been made to image the pancreas, take the required images in the designated areas and add "AREA" to the labeling.

PART III

Right Kidney • Longitudinal Image

25. Long axis image of the right kidney.

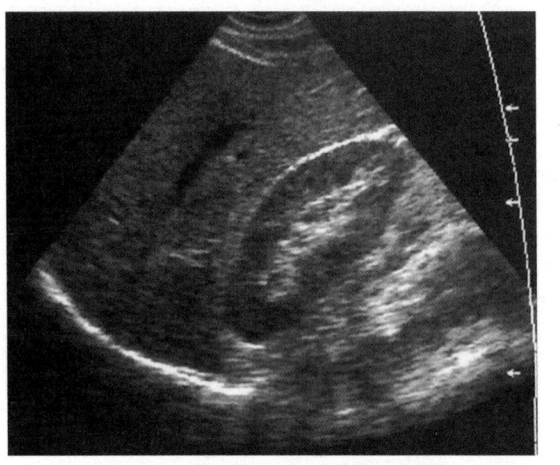

Labeled: **RT KID SAG LONG AXIS**

SCANNING TIP: Take an additional image of the superior and/or inferior poles if they are not clearly represented on the long axis image. Label accordingly.

Right Kidney • Axial Image

26. Axial image of the right kidney midportion to include the hilum.

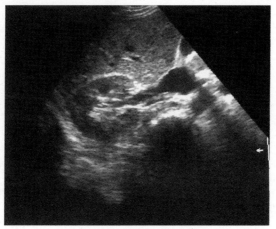

Labeled: **RT KID TRV MID**

Left Kidney • Longitudinal Image

27. Long axis image of the left kidney.

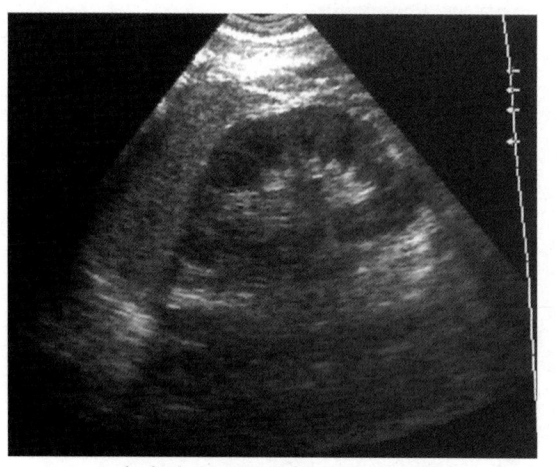

Labeled: **LT KID COR LONG AXIS**

SCANNING TIP: Take an additional image of the superior and/or inferior poles if they are not clearly represented on the long axis image. Label accordingly.

Left Kidney • Axial Image

28. Axial image of the left kidney midportion to include the hilum.

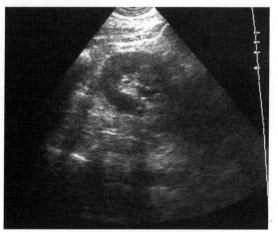

Labeled: **LT KID LT TRV MID**

Spleen • Longitudinal Images

29. Long axis image of the spleen.

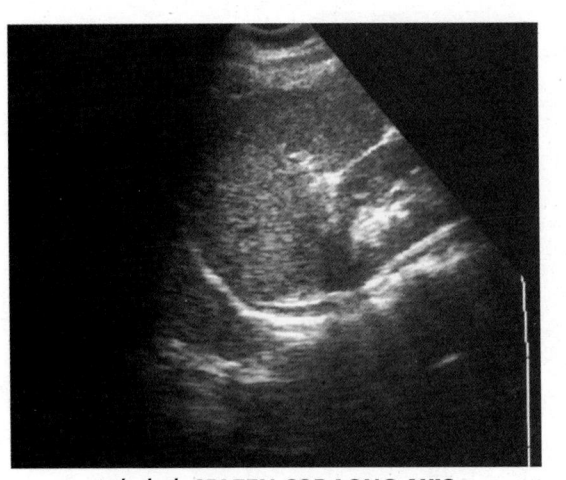

Labeled: **SPLEEN COR LONG AXIS**

SCANNING TIP: If the adjacent pleural space and a portion of the left kidney were adequately demonstrated on number 29, numbers 30 and/or 31 may be omitted.

30. Superior longitudinal image of the spleen to include the adjacent pleural space.

31. Inferior longitudinal image of the spleen to include part of the left kidney for parenchyma comparison.

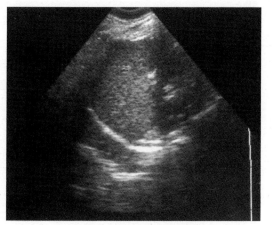

Labeled: **SPLEEN COR SUP**

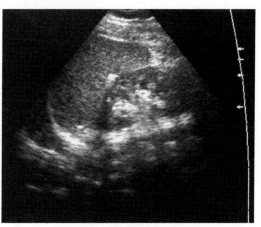

Labeled: **SPLEEN COR INF**

Spleen • Axial Images

32. Axial image of the spleen to include both anterior and posterior margins.

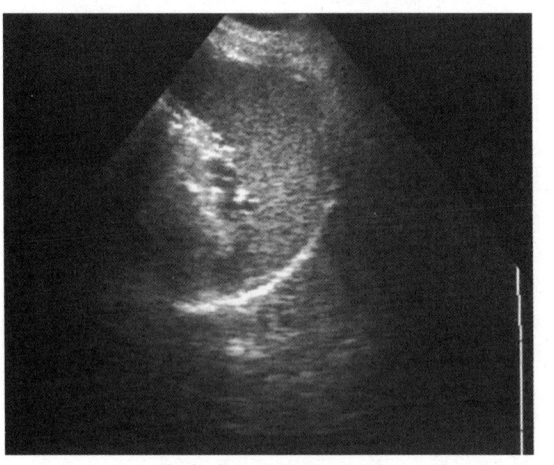

Labeled: **SPLEEN LT TRV**

SCANNING TIP: If the anterior and posterior margins were adequately demonstrated on number 32, numbers 33 and/or 34 may be omitted.

33. Axial image of the spleen to include both anterior margin and splenic hilum.

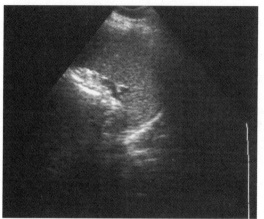

Labeled: **SPLEEN LT TRV ANT**

34. Axial image of the spleen to include the posterior margin.

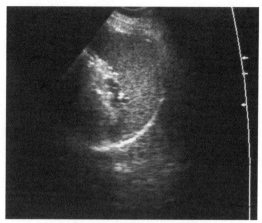

Labeled: **SPLEEN LT TRV POST**

SECTION TWO ▪ Image Protocols for Limited Sonographic Studies of the Abdomen

- Extensive images of the area(s) of interest:
  - Aorta Study With Limited Abdomen
  - Inferior Vena Cava Study With Limited Abdomen
  - Right Upper Quadrant Study With Limited Abdomen
  - Gallbladder and Biliary Tract Study With Limited Abdomen
  - Pancreas Study With Limited Abdomen
  - Renal Study With Limited Abdomen
  - Spleen Study With Limited Abdomen

Criteria

- Begin studies with a survey of abdominal structures in at least 2 scanning planes.
- Do not share study results with the patient. Legally, only physicians can give diagnoses.

Aorta Study With Limited Abdomen

Aorta • Longitudinal Images

1. Longitudinal image of the proximal aorta (inferior to the diaphragm, superior to the celiac trunk).

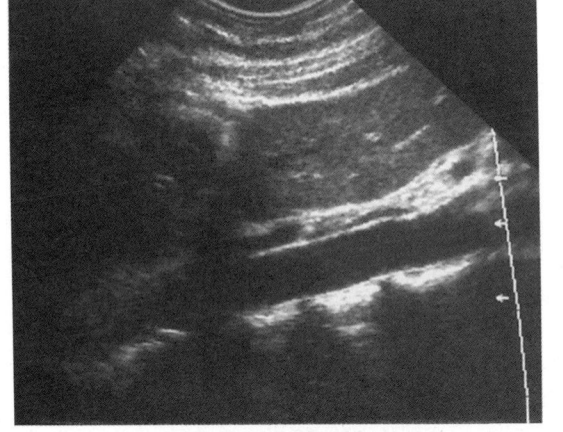

Labeled: **AORTA SAG PROX**

2. Longitudinal image of the middle aorta (inferior to the celiac trunk along the length of the superior mesenteric artery).

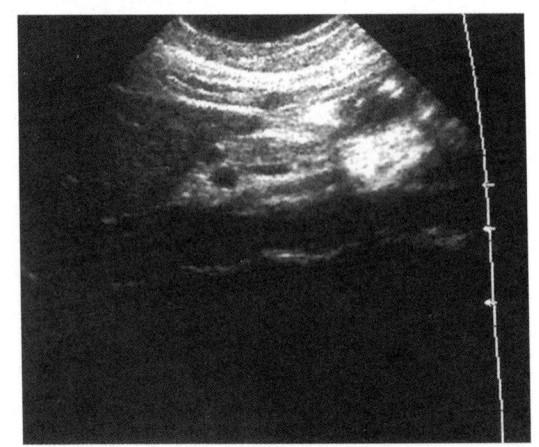

Labeled: **AORTA SAG MID**

3. Longitudinal image of the distal aorta (inferior to the superior mesenteric artery, superior to the bifurcation).

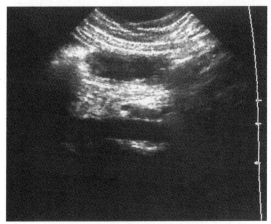

Labeled: **AORTA SAG DISTAL**

4. Longitudinal image of the aorta bifurcation (common iliac arteries).

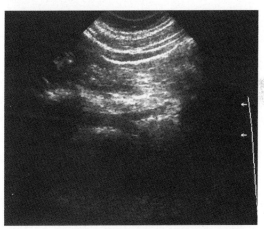

Labeled: **AORTA SAG BIF RT or LT OBL or AORTA LT COR BIF**

PART III

Aorta • Axial Images

5. Axial image of the proximal aorta (inferior to the diaphragm, superior to the celiac trunk) *with anterior to posterior measurement* (calipers) *outside wall to outside wall*).

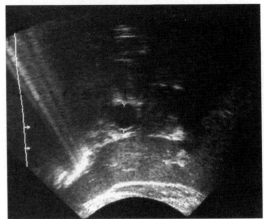

Labeled: AORTA TRV PROX

6. Same image as number 5, *without measurement calipers.*

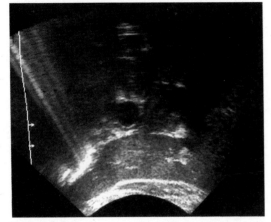

Labeled: AORTA TRV PROX

7. Axial image of the middle aorta (inferior to the celiac trunk along the length of the superior mesenteric artery) *with anterior to posterior measurement* (calipers outside wall to outside wall).

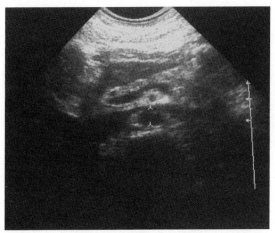

Labeled: **AORTA TRV MID**

8. Same image as number 7, *without measurement calipers.*

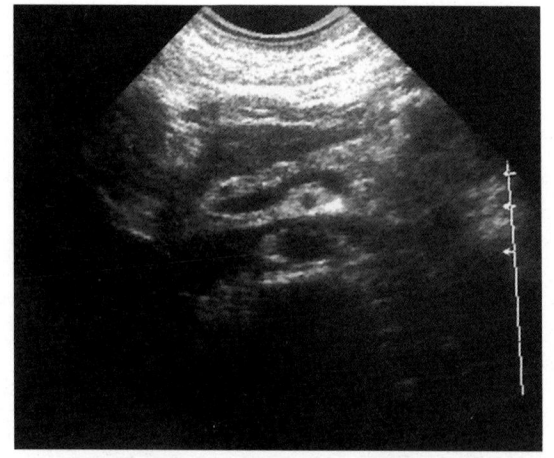

Labeled: **AORTA TRV MID**

SCANNING TIP: If the renal arteries were represented on number 7, numbers 9 and/or 10 may be omitted.

9. Longitudinal image of the right renal artery.

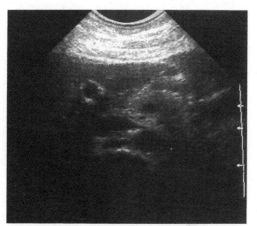

Labeled: **RT RENAL ART TRV**

10. Longitudinal image of the left renal artery.

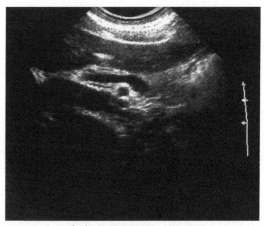

Labeled: **LT RENAL ART TRV**

PART III

11. Axial image of the distal aorta (inferior to the superior mesenteric artery, superior to the bifurcation) *with anterior to posterior measurement* (calipers outside wall to outside wall).

12. Same image as number 11, *without measurement calipers.*

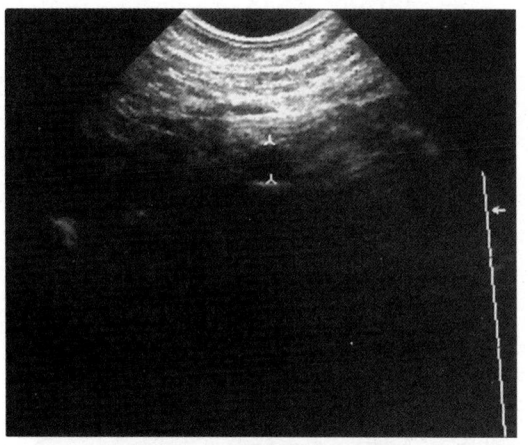

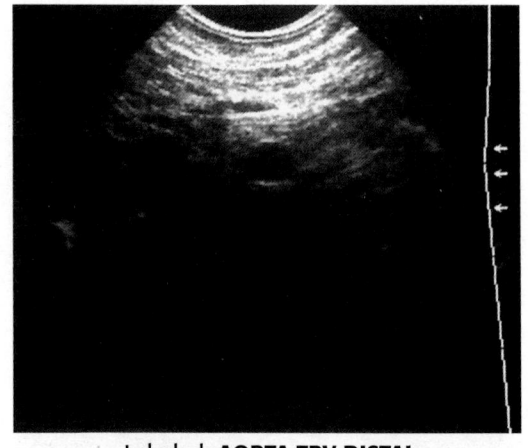

Labeled: **AORTA TRV DISTAL**

Labeled: **AORTA TRV DISTAL**

13. Axial image of aorta bifurcation (common iliac arteries).

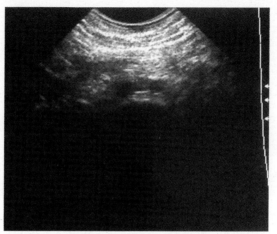

Labeled: **AORTA TRV BIF**

Inferior Vena Cava Study With Limited Abdomen

Inferior Vena Cava • Longitudinal Images

1. Longitudinal image of the distal inferior vena cava (IVC) to include the diaphragm and hepatic vein(s).

2. Longitudinal image of the middle IVC at the level of the head of the pancreas.

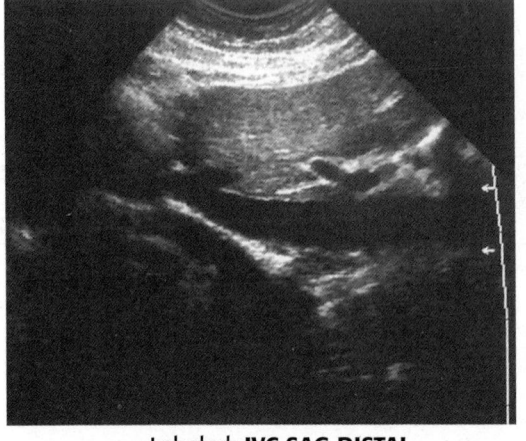

Labeled: **IVC SAG DISTAL**

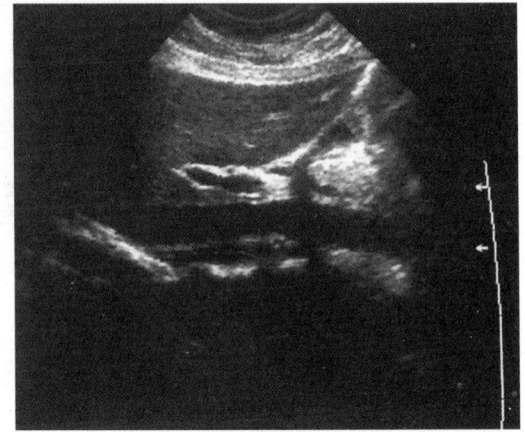

Labeled: **IVC SAG MID**

3. Longitudinal image of the proximal IVC.

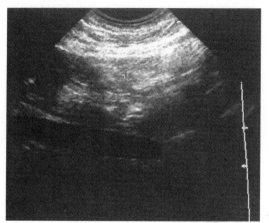

Labeled: **IVC SAG PROX**

4. Longitudinal image of the IVC bifurcation (common iliac veins).

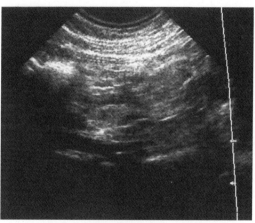

Labeled: **IVC SAG BIF RT** or **LT OBL** or **IVC RT COR BIF**

Inferior Vena Cava • Axial Images

5. Axial image of the distal IVC to include the hepatic veins.

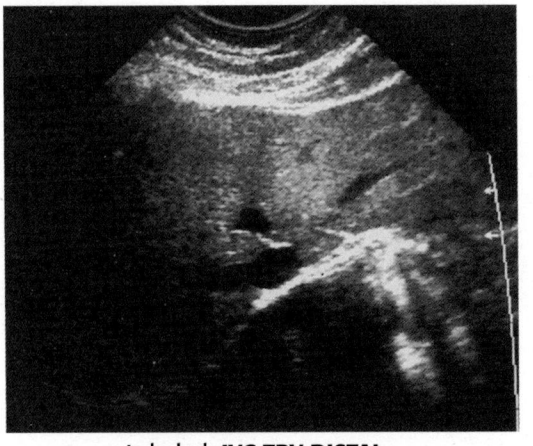

Labeled: **IVC TRV DISTAL**

6. Axial image of the IVC at the level of the renal veins.

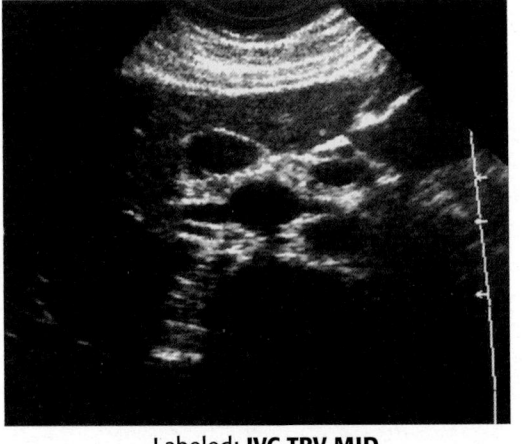

Labeled: **IVC TRV MID**

7. Axial image of the proximal IVC.

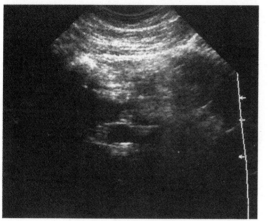

Labeled: **IVC TRV PROX**

8. Axial image of the IVC bifurcation (common iliac veins).

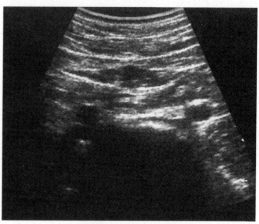

Labeled: **IVC TRV BIF**

Right Upper Quadrant Study With Limited Abdomen

Liver • Longitudinal Images

1. Longitudinal image of the left lobe of the liver to include the inferior margin and the aorta.

2. Longitudinal image of the left lobe of the liver to include the diaphragm and caudate lobe.

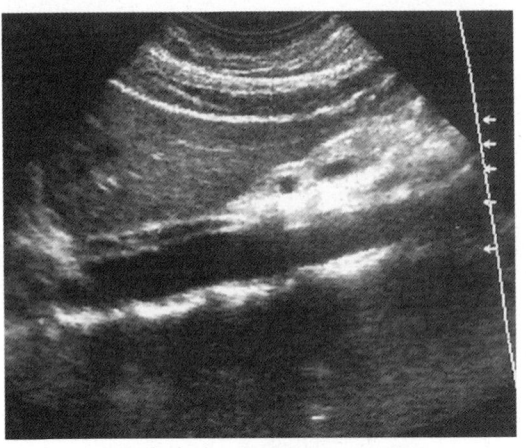

Labeled: **LIVER SAG LT LOBE**

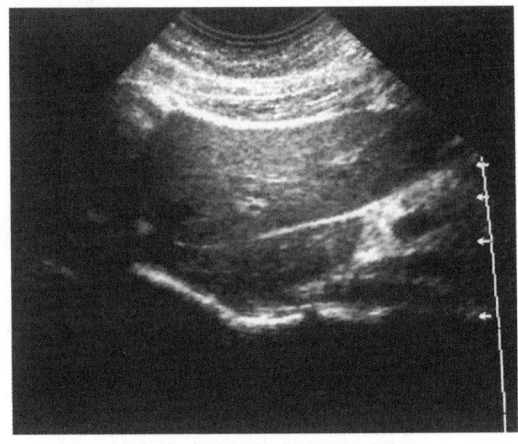

Labeled: **LIVER SAG LT LOBE**

3. Longitudinal image of the right lobe of the liver to include the IVC where it passes through the liver.

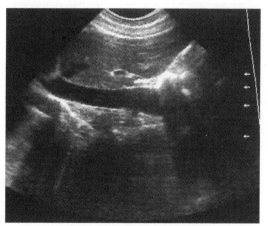

Labeled: **LIVER SAG RT LOBE**

4. Longitudinal image of the right lobe of the liver to include the main lobar fissure, gallbladder, and portal vein.

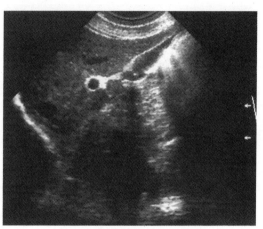

Labeled: **LIVER SAG RT LOBE**

5. Longitudinal image of the right lobe of the liver to include part of the right kidney for parenchyma comparison.

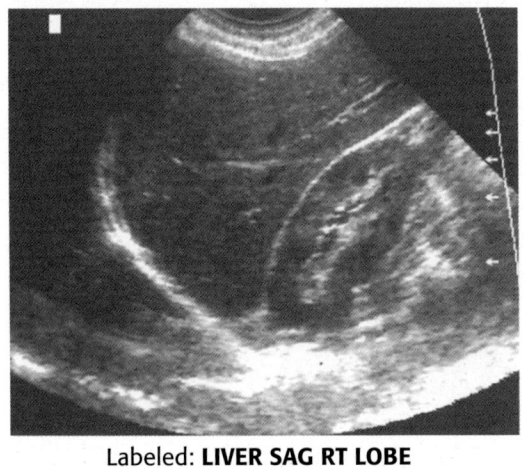

Labeled: **LIVER SAG RT LOBE**

6. Longitudinal image of the right lobe of the liver to include the dome and adjacent pleural space.

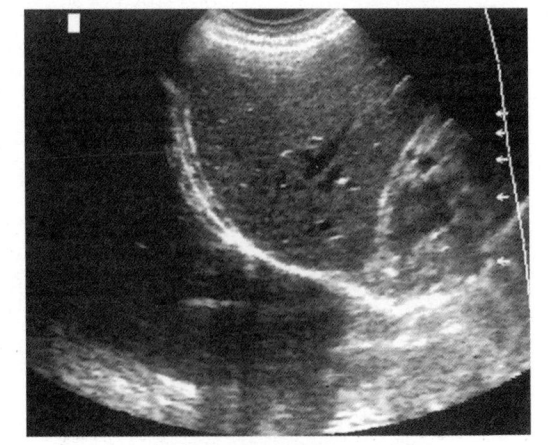

Labeled: **LIVER SAG RT LOBE**

Liver • Axial Images

7. Axial image of the left lobe of the liver to include its lateral margin.

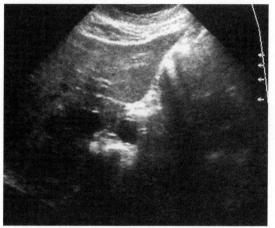

Labeled: **LIVER TRV LT LOBE**

8. Axial image of the left lobe of the liver to include the ligamentum teres.

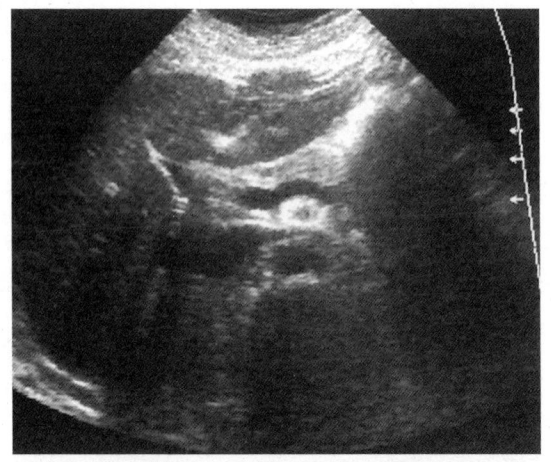

Labeled: **LIVER TRV LT LOBE**

SCANNING TIP: Depending on liver size and shape, it may be possible to document an axial image of the left lobe that includes both the lateral margin and ligamentum teres. If so, label the image as follows:
LIVER TRV LT LOBE

9. Axial image of the right lobe of the liver to include the hepatic veins.

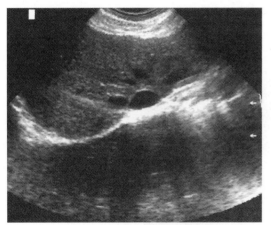

Labeled: **LIVER TRV RT LOBE**

10. Axial image of the right lobe of the liver to include the right and left branches of the portal vein.

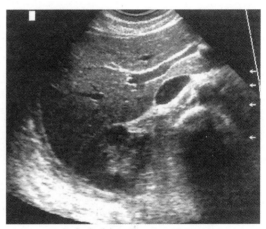

Labeled: **LIVER TRV RT LOBE**

11. Axial image of the right lobe of the liver to include the right lateral inferior lobe.

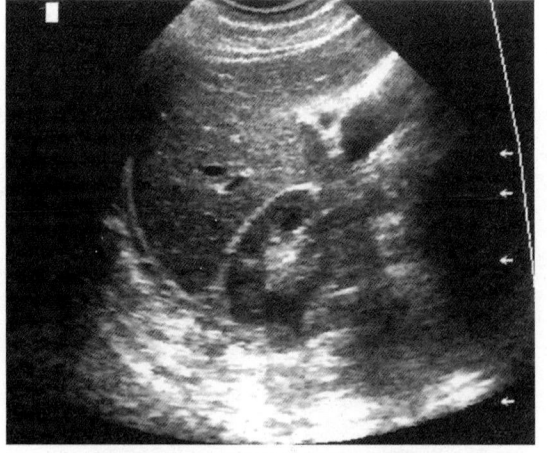

Labeled: **LIVER TRV RT LOBE**

12. Axial image of the right lobe of the liver to include the dome and adjacent pleural space.

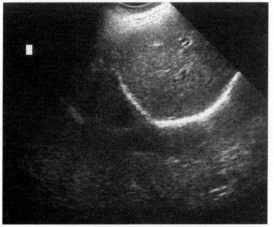

Labeled: **LIVER TRV RT LOBE**

SCANNING TIP: Routine measurements of the liver are not required.

Inferior Vena Cava • Longitudinal Image

SCANNING TIP: The images of the IVC may be included with the liver images if the IVC is well visualized.

13. Longitudinal image of the distal and middle IVC.

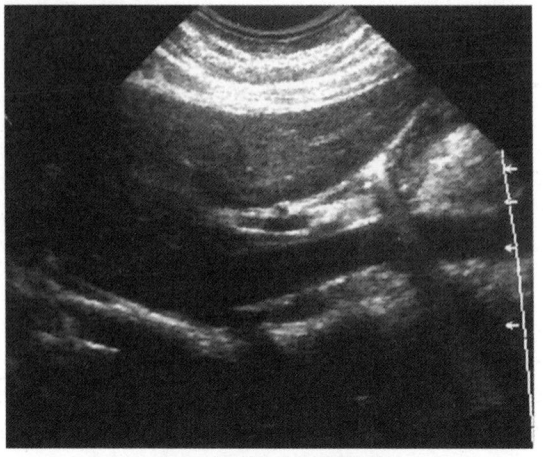

Labeled: **IVC SAG DISTAL**

Inferior Vena Cava • Axial Image

14. Axial image of the distal IVC to include the hepatic veins.

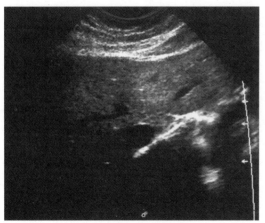

Labeled: **IVC TRV DISTAL**

Gallbladder and Biliary Tract • First Position
Gallbladder • Longitudinal Images

15. Long axis image of the gallbladder.

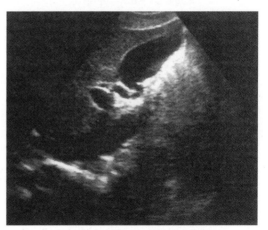

Labeled: **GB SAG LONG AXIS**

16. Longitudinal image of the gallbladder fundus and body.

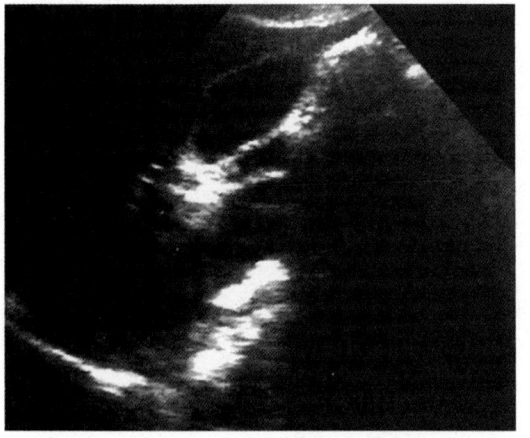

Labeled: **GB SAG FUNDUS/BODY**

17. Longitudinal image of the gallbladder neck.

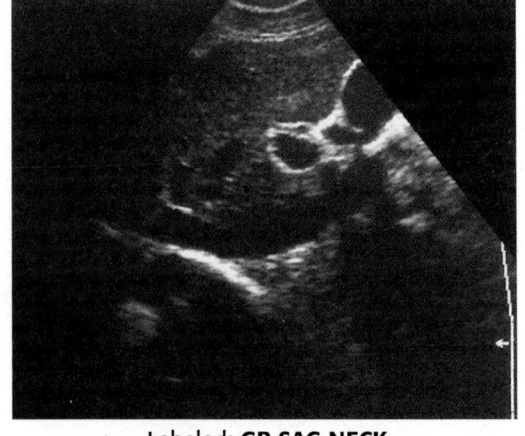

Labeled: **GB SAG NECK**

Gallbladder • Axial Images

18. Axial image of the gallbladder fundus.

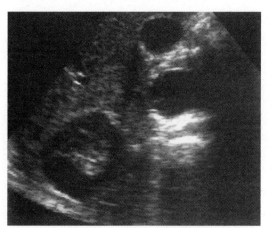

Labeled: **GB TRV FUNDUS**

19. Axial image of the gallbladder body.

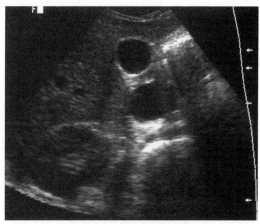

Labeled: **GB TRV BODY**

20. Axial image of the gallbladder neck.

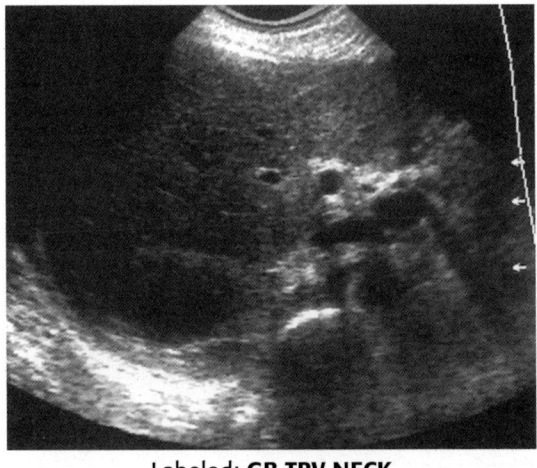

Labeled: **GB TRV NECK**

Biliary Tract • Longitudinal Images

SCANNING TIP: Biliary tract images may be magnified to aid interpretation.

SCANNING TIP: The common hepatic duct (CHD) image may be omitted if the CHD was visualized on the gallbladder long axis image.

SCANNING TIP: Biliary tract images may be taken in the second patient position if they were better visualized there during the survey.

21. Longitudinal image of the CHD.

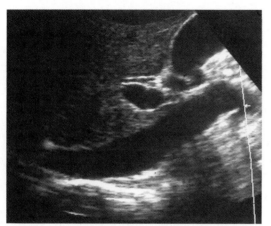

Labeled: **SAG CHD**

22. Longitudinal image of the common bile duct *with anterior to posterior measurement at the widest margins of the lumen.*

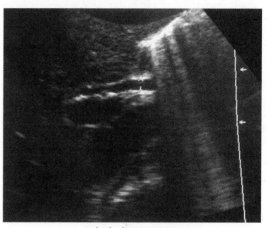

Labeled: **SAG CBD**

23. Same image as number 22 *without measurement calipers*.

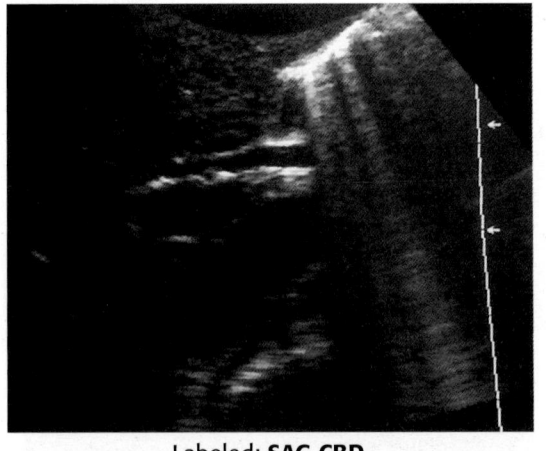

Labeled: **SAG CBD**

Gallbladder and Biliary Tract • Second Position
Gallbladder • Longitudinal Image

24. Long axis image of the gallbladder.

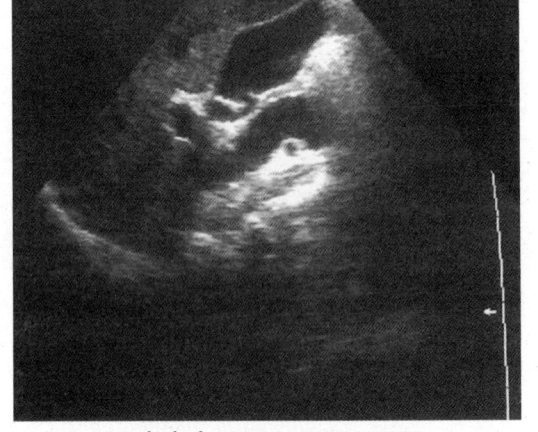

Labeled: **GB SAG LONG AXIS**

Gallbladder • Axial Image

25. Axial image of the gallbladder fundus.

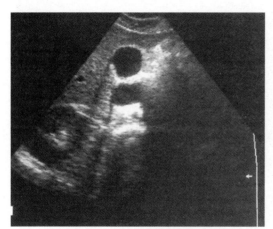

Labeled: **GB TRV FUNDUS**

Pancreas • Longitudinal Images

26. Long axis image of the pancreas to include as much head, uncinate, neck, body, tail, and pancreatic duct as possible.

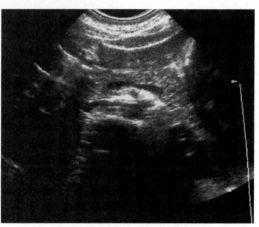

Labeled: **PANC TRV LONG AXIS**

27. Longitudinal image of the pancreas head to include the uncinate process and common bile duct (if bile filled).

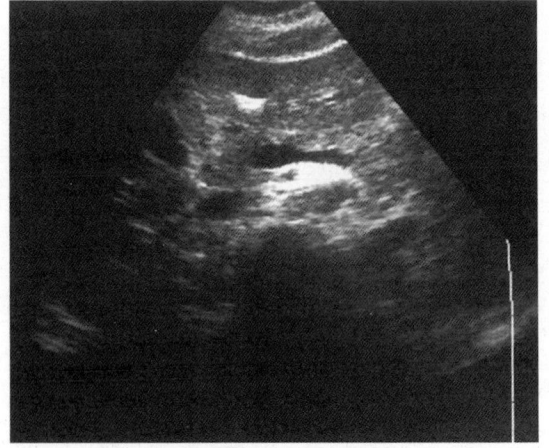

Labeled: **PANC TRV HEAD**

Pancreas • Axial Image

28. Axial image of the pancreas head to include the common bile duct (if bile filled).

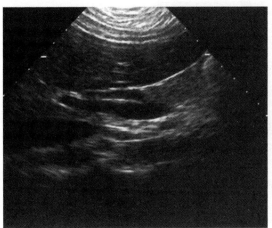

Labeled: **PANC SAG HEAD**

SCANNING TIP: In some cases, a portion or all of the pancreas cannot be visualized because of overlying bowel gas and the patient cannot be given fluids to displace the gas. When this occurs, and every effort has been made to image the pancreas, take the required images in the designated areas and add "AREA" to the labeling.

Right Kidney • Longitudinal Image

29. Long axis image of the right kidney.

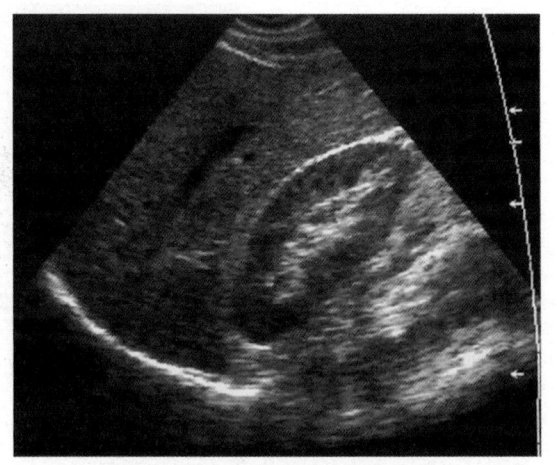

Labeled: **RT KID SAG LONG AXIS**

SCANNING TIP: Take an additional image of the superior and/or inferior poles if they are not clearly represented on the long axis image. Label accordingly.

Right Kidney • Axial Image

30. Axial image of the right kidney midportion to include the hilum.

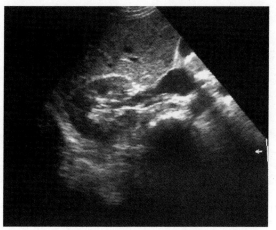

Labeled: **RT KID TRV MID**

PART III

Gallbladder and Biliary Tract Study With Limited Abdomen

Liver • Longitudinal Images

1. Longitudinal image of the left lobe of the liver to include the inferior margin and the aorta.

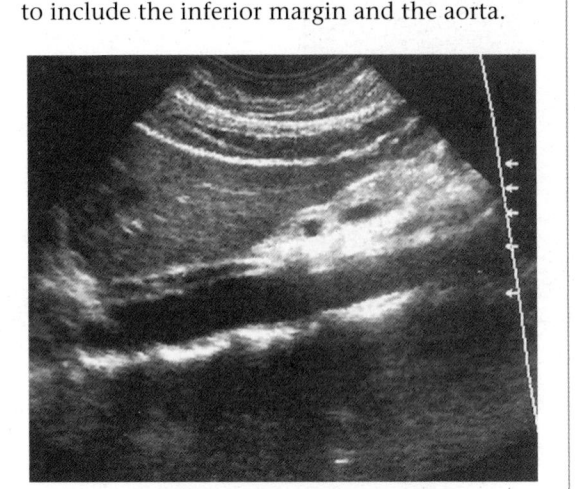

Labeled: **LIVER SAG LT LOBE**

2. Longitudinal image of the left lobe of the liver to include the diaphragm and caudate lobe.

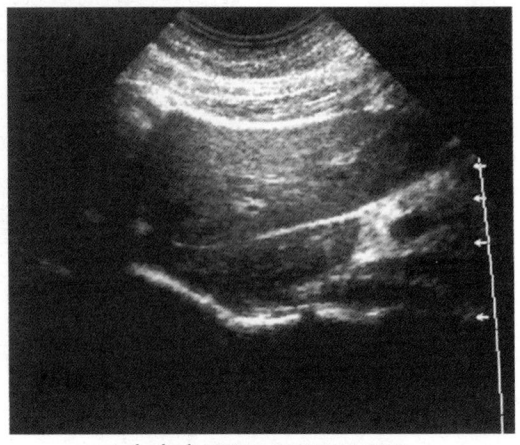

Labeled: **LIVER SAG LT LOBE**

3. Longitudinal image of the right lobe of the liver to include the IVC where it passes through the liver.

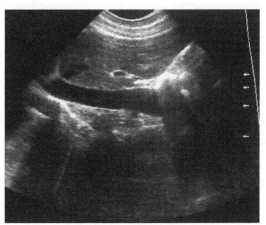

Labeled: **LIVER SAG RT LOBE**

4. Longitudinal image of the right lobe of the liver to include the main lobar fissure, gallbladder, and portal vein.

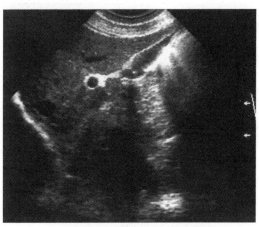

Labeled: **LIVER SAG RT LOBE**

5. Longitudinal image of the right lobe of the liver to include part of the right kidney for parenchyma comparison.

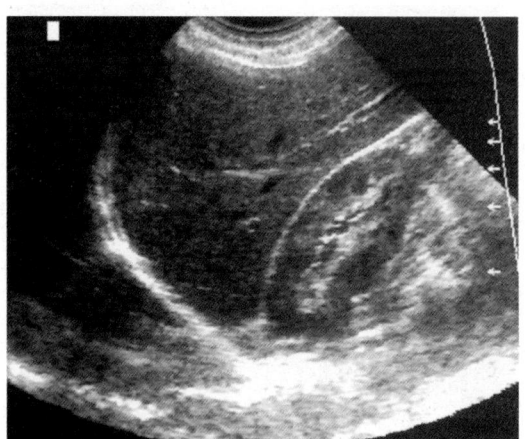

Labeled: **LIVER SAG RT LOBE**

6. Longitudinal image of the right lobe of the liver to include the dome and adjacent pleural space.

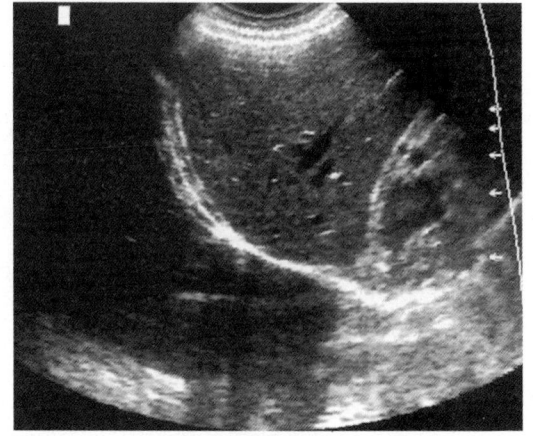

Labeled: **LIVER SAG RT LOBE**

Liver • Axial Images

7. Axial image of the left lobe of the liver to include its lateral margin.

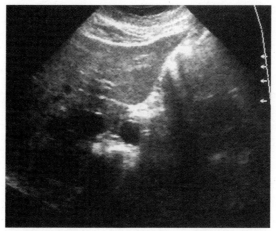

Labeled: **LIVER TRV LT LOBE**

PART III

8. Axial image of the left lobe of the liver to include the ligamentum teres.

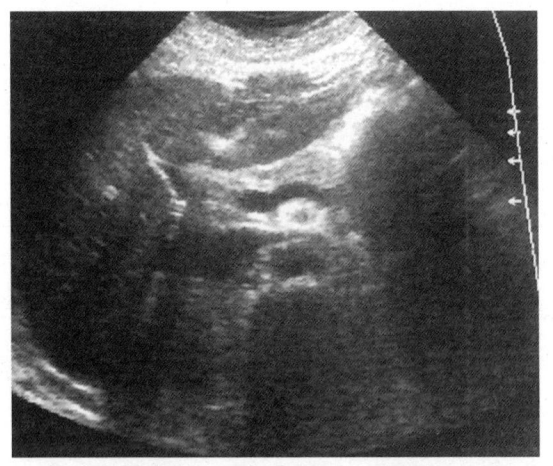

Labeled: **LIVER TRV LT LOBE**

SCANNING TIP: Depending on liver size and shape, it may be possible to document an axial image of the left lobe that includes both the lateral margin and ligamentum teres. If so, label the image as follows:
LIVER TRV LT LOBE

9. Axial image of the right lobe of the liver to include the hepatic veins.

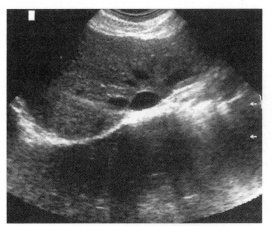

Labeled: **LIVER TRV RT LOBE**

10. Axial image of the right lobe of the liver to include the right and left branches of the portal vein.

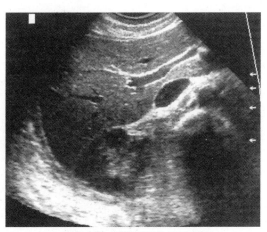

Labeled: **LIVER TRV RT LOBE**

PART III

11. Axial image of the right lobe of the liver to include the right lateral inferior lobe.

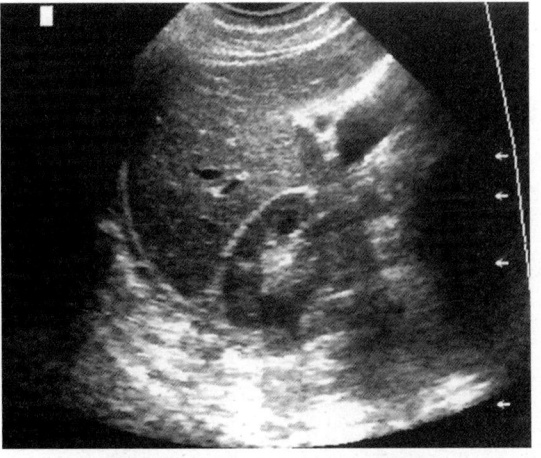

Labeled: **LIVER TRV RT LOBE**

12. Axial image of the right lobe of the liver to include the dome and adjacent pleural space.

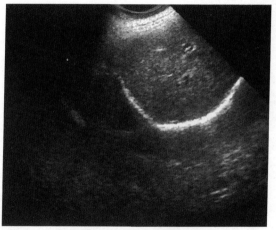

Labeled: **LIVER TRV RT LOBE**

SCANNING TIP: Routine measurements of the liver are not required.

PART III

Gallbladder and Biliary Tract • First Position

> **SCANNING TIP:** When the gallbladder and biliary tract are the areas of interest, they are routinely surveyed in 2 different patient positions and the gallbladder is documented in both positions.

Gallbladder • Longitudinal Images

13. Long axis image of the gallbladder.

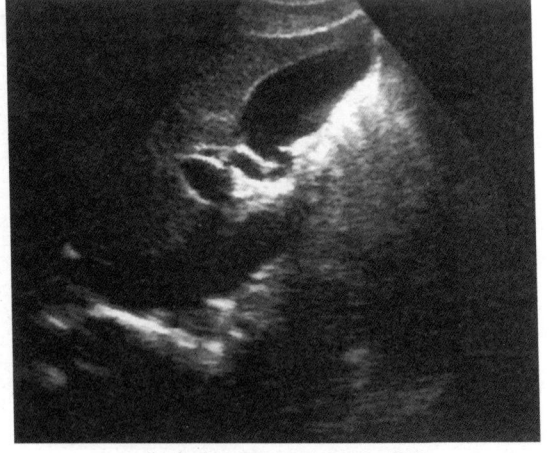

Labeled: **GB SAG LONG AXIS**

14. Longitudinal image of the gallbladder fundus and body.

15. Longitudinal image of the gallbladder neck.

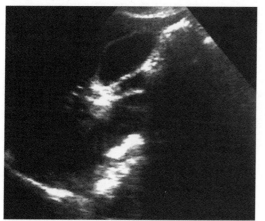

Labeled: **GB SAG FUNDUS/BODY**

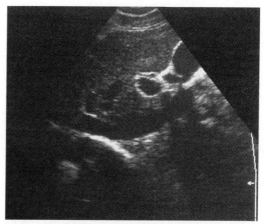

Labeled: **GB SAG NECK**

PART III

Gallbladder • Axial Images

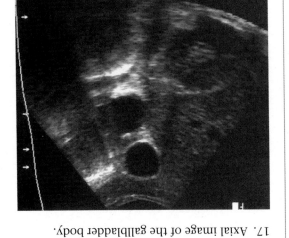

17. Axial image of the gallbladder body.

Labeled: **SAG CHD**

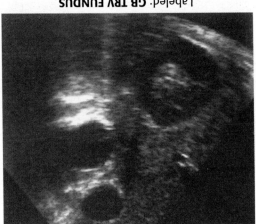

16. Axial image of the gallbladder fundus.

Labeled: **GB TRV FUNDUS**

18. Axial image of the gallbladder neck.

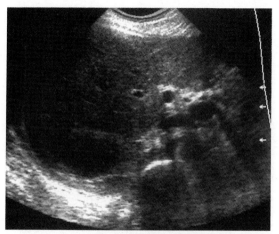

Labeled: **GB TRV NECK**

Biliary Tract • Longitudinal Images

SCANNING TIP: Biliary tract images may be magnified to aid interpretation.

SCANNING TIP: The CHD image may be omitted if the CHD was visualized on the gallbladder long axis image.

SCANNING TIP: Biliary tract images may be taken in the second patient position if they were better visualized there during the survey.

19. Longitudinal image of the CHD.

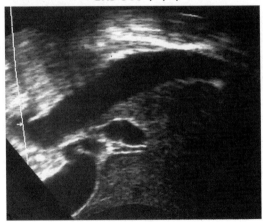

Labeled: **SAG CHD**

20. Longitudinal image of the common bile duct with anterior to posterior measurement at the widest margins of the lumen.

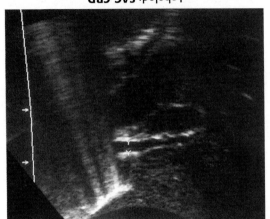

Labeled: **SAG CBD**

21. Same image as number 20 *without measurement calipers.*

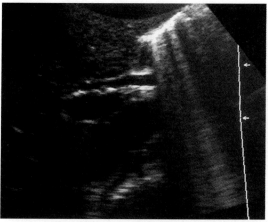

Labeled: **SAG CBD**

Gallbladder and Biliary Tract • Second Position
Gallbladder • Longitudinal Image

SCANNING TIP: Biliary tract images may be magnified to aid interpretation.

SCANNING TIP: The CHD image may be omitted if the CHD was visualized on the gallbladder long axis image.

SCANNING TIP: Biliary tract images may be taken in the second patient position if they were better visualized there during the survey.

Gallbladder • *Axial Image*

22. Long axis image of the gallbladder.

23. Axial image of the gallbladder fundus.

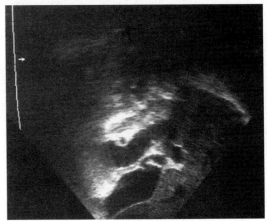

Labeled: **GB SAG LONG AXIS**

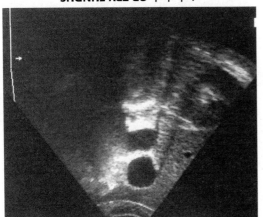

Labeled: **GB TRV FUNDUS**

Pancreas • Longitudinal Images

24. Long axis image of the pancreas to include as much head, uncinate, neck, body, tail, and pancreatic duct as possible.

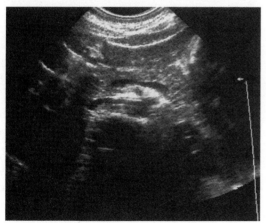

Labeled: **PANC TRV LONG AXIS**

25. Longitudinal image of the pancreas head to include the uncinate process and common bile duct (if bile filled).

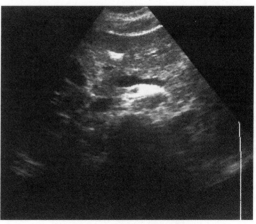

Labeled: **PANC TRV HEAD**

PART III

Pancreas • Axial Image

26. Axial image of the pancreas head to include the common bile duct (if bile filled).

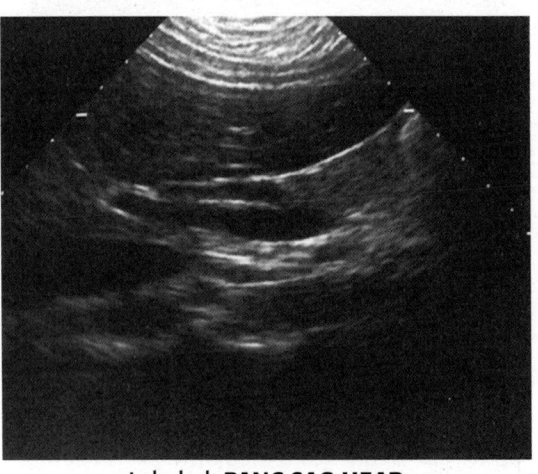

Labeled: **PANC SAG HEAD**

SCANNING TIP: In some cases, a portion or all of the pancreas cannot be visualized because of overlying bowel gas and the patient cannot be given fluids to displace the gas. When this occurs, and every effort has been made to image the pancreas, take the required images in the designated areas and add "AREA" to the labeling.

Pancreas Study With Limited Abdomen

Liver • Longitudinal Images

1. Longitudinal image of the left lobe of the liver to include the inferior margin and the aorta.

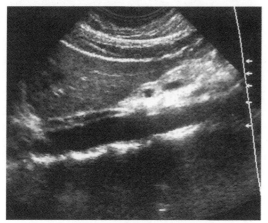

Labeled: **LIVER SAG LT LOBE**

2. Longitudinal image of the left lobe of the liver to include the diaphragm and caudate lobe.

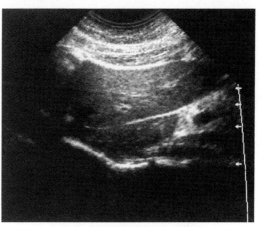

Labeled: **LIVER SAG LT LOBE**

PART III

3. Longitudinal image of the right lobe of the liver to include the IVC where it passes through the liver.

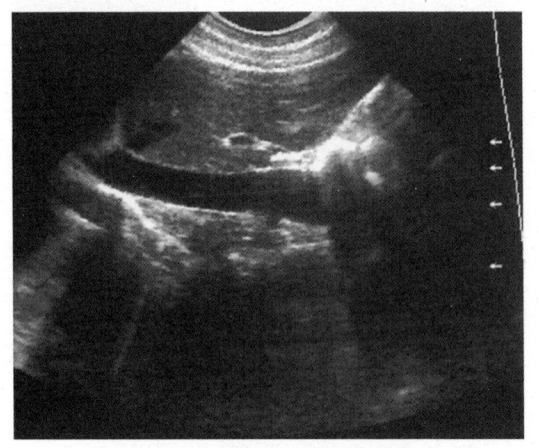

Labeled: **LIVER SAG RT LOBE**

4. Longitudinal image of the right lobe of the liver to include the main lobar fissure, gallbladder, and portal vein.

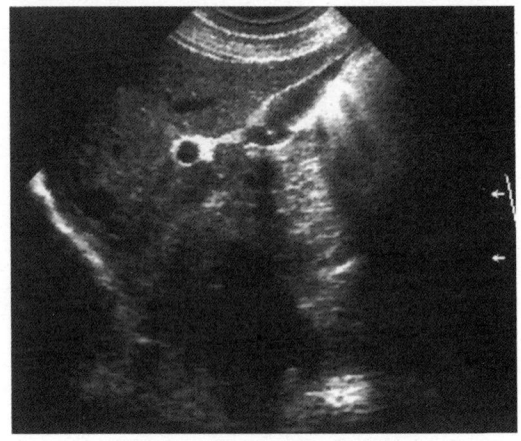

Labeled: **LIVER SAG RT LOBE**

5. Longitudinal image of the right lobe of the liver to include part of the right kidney for parenchyma comparison.

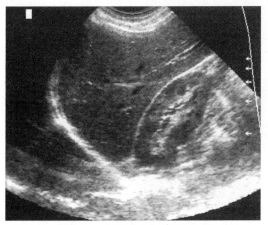

Labeled: **LIVER SAG RT LOBE**

6. Longitudinal image of the right lobe of the liver to include the dome and adjacent pleural space.

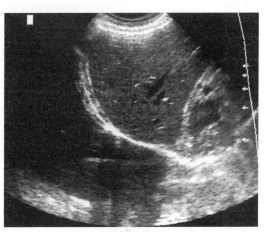

Labeled: **LIVER SAG RT LOBE**

Liver • Axial Images

7. Axial image of the left lobe of the liver to include its lateral margin.

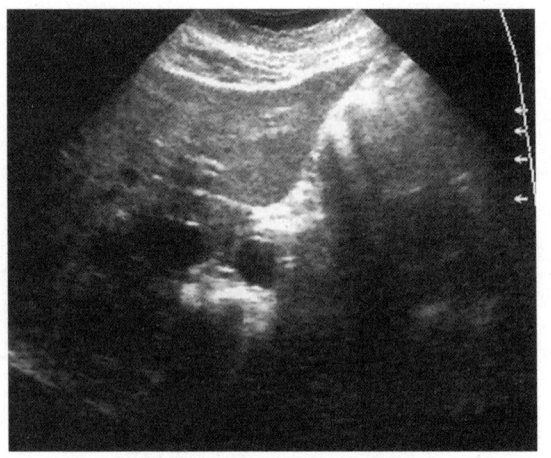

Labeled: **LIVER TRV LT LOBE**

8. Axial image of the left lobe of the liver to include the ligamentum teres.

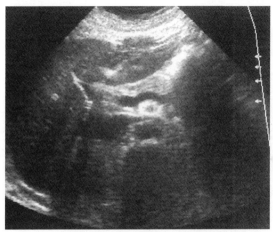

Labeled: **LIVER TRV LT LOBE**

SCANNING TIP: Depending on liver size and shape, it may be possible to document an axial image of the left lobe that includes both the lateral margin and ligamentum teres. If so, label the image as follows:
LIVER TRV LT LOBE

9. Axial image of the right lobe of the liver to include the hepatic veins.

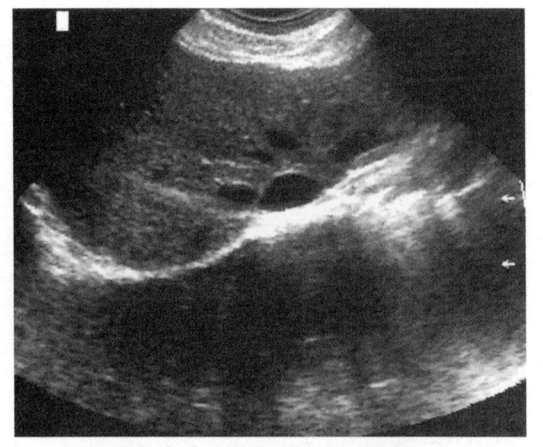

Labeled: **LIVER TRV RT LOBE**

10. Axial image of the right lobe of the liver to include the right and left branches of the portal vein.

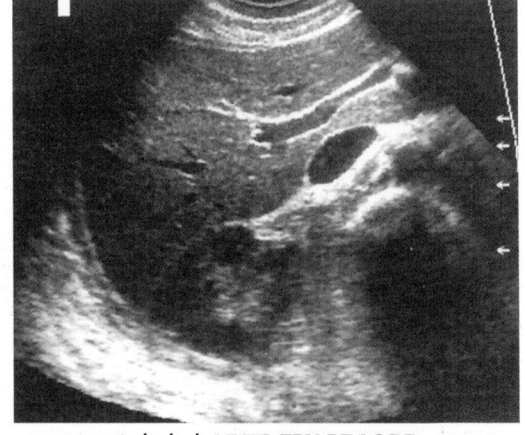

Labeled: **LIVER TRV RT LOBE**

11. Axial image of the right lobe of the liver to include the right lateral inferior lobe.

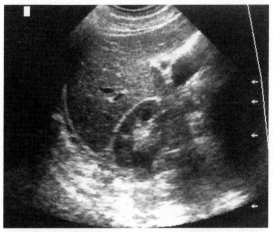

Labeled: **LIVER TRV RT LOBE**

12. Axial image of the right lobe of the liver to include the dome and adjacent pleural space.

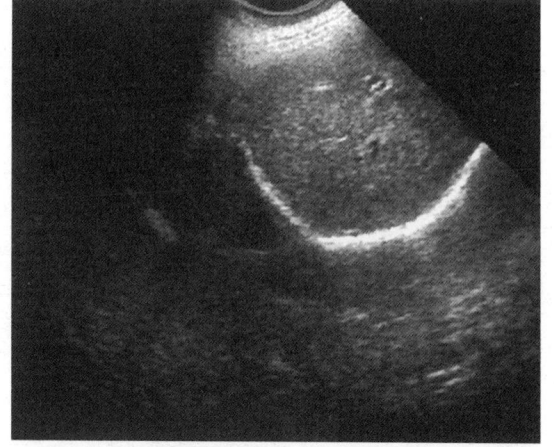

Labeled: **LIVER TRV RT LOBE**

SCANNING TIP: Routine measurements of the liver are not required.

Gallbladder • Longitudinal Image

13. Long axis image of the gallbladder.

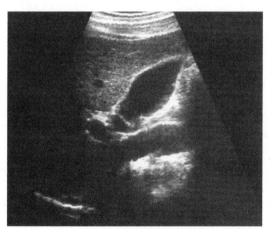

Labeled: **GB SAG LONG AXIS**

Gallbladder • Axial Image

14. Axial image of the gallbladder fundus.

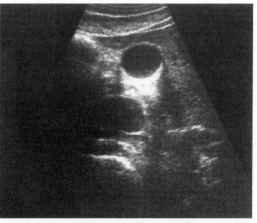

Labeled: **GB TRV FUNDUS**

Biliary Tract • Longitudinal Images

SCANNING TIP: Biliary tract images may be magnified to aid interpretation.

SCANNING TIP: The CHD image may be omitted if the CHD was visualized on the gallbladder long axis image.

15. Longitudinal image of the CHD.

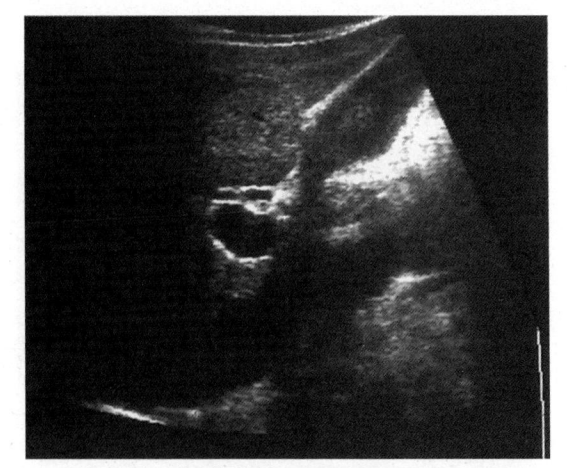

Labeled: **SAG CHD**

16. Longitudinal image of the common bile duct *with anterior to posterior measurement at the widest margins of the lumen.*

17. Same image as number 16 *without measurement calipers.*

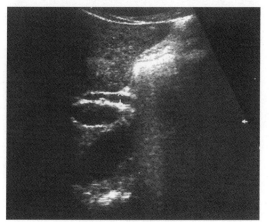

Labeled: **SAG CBD**

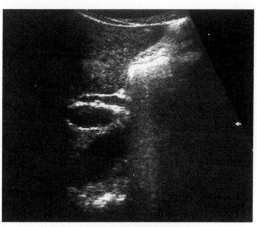

Labeled: **SAG CBD**

PART III

Pancreas • Longitudinal Images

18. Long axis image of the pancreas to include as much head, uncinate, neck, body, tail, and pancreatic duct as possible.

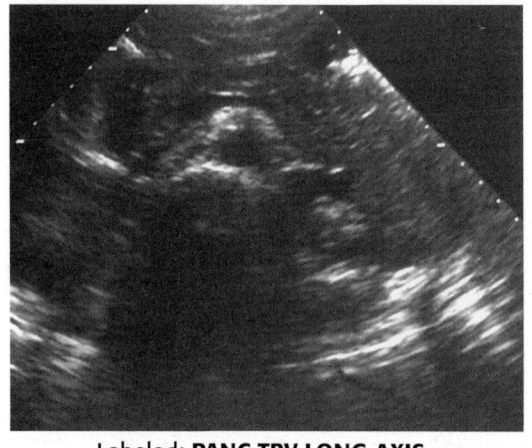

Labeled: **PANC TRV LONG AXIS**

19. Longitudinal image of the pancreas body and neck to include the splenic vein.

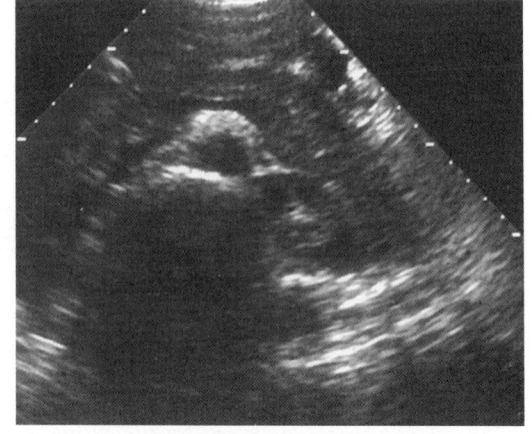

Labeled: **PANC TRV BODY/NECK**

20. Longitudinal image of the pancreas tail.

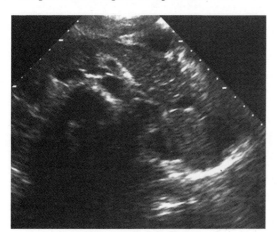

Labeled: **PANC TRV TAIL**

21. Longitudinal image of the pancreas head to include the uncinate process and common bile duct (if bile filled).

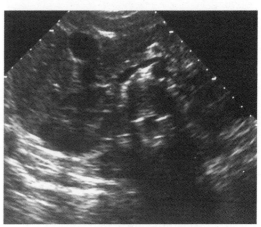

Labeled: **PANC TRV HEAD**

PART III

Pancreas • Axial Images

22. Axial image of the pancreas head to include the common bile duct (if bile filled).

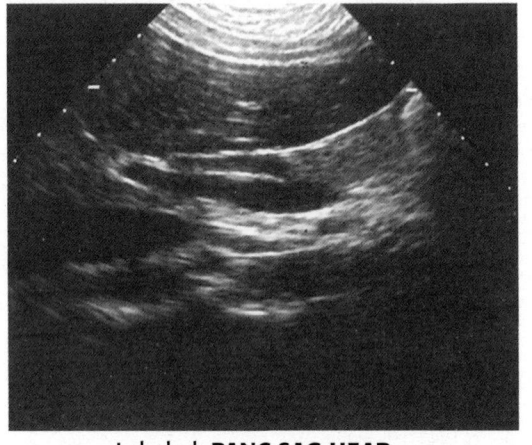

Labeled: **PANC SAG HEAD**

23. Axial image of the pancreas neck and uncinate process to include the superior mesenteric vein.

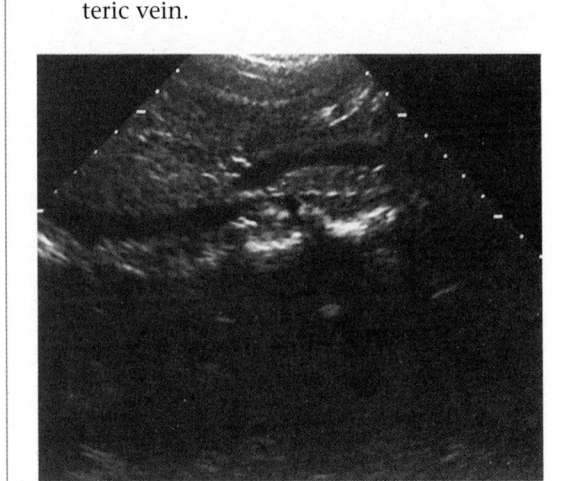

Labeled: **PANC SAG NECK/UNCINATE**

24. Axial image of the pancreas body to include the splenic vein.

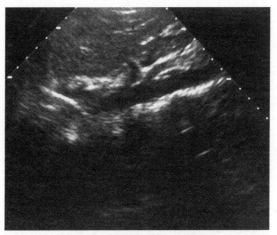

Labeled: **PANC SAG BODY**

25. Axial image of the pancreas tail.

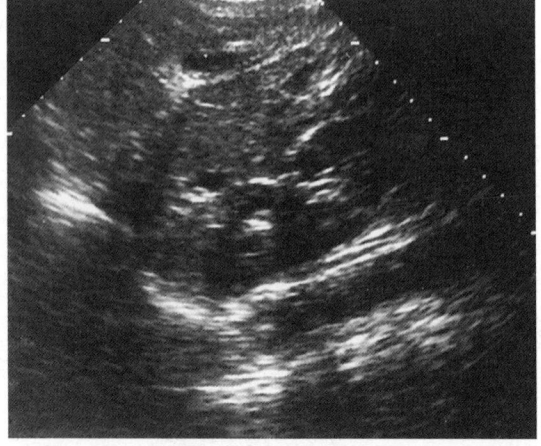

Labeled: **PANC SAG TAIL**

SCANNING TIP: In some cases, a portion or all of the pancreas cannot be visualized because of overlying bowel gas and the patient cannot be given fluids to displace the gas. When this occurs, and every effort has been made to image the pancreas, take the required images in the designated areas and add "AREA" to the labeling.

Renal Study With Limited Abdomen

Right Kidney • Longitudinal Images

1. Long axis image of the right kidney *with superior to inferior measurement.*

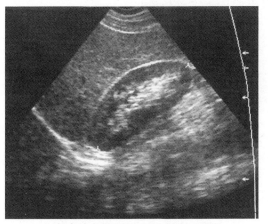

Labeled: **RT KID SAG LONG AXIS**

2. Same image as number 1 *without measurement calipers.*

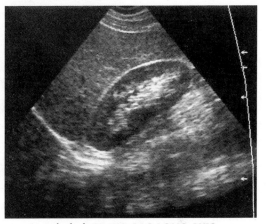

Labeled: **RT KID SAG LONG AXIS**

PART III

3. Long axis image of the right kidney *with superior to inferior measurement.*

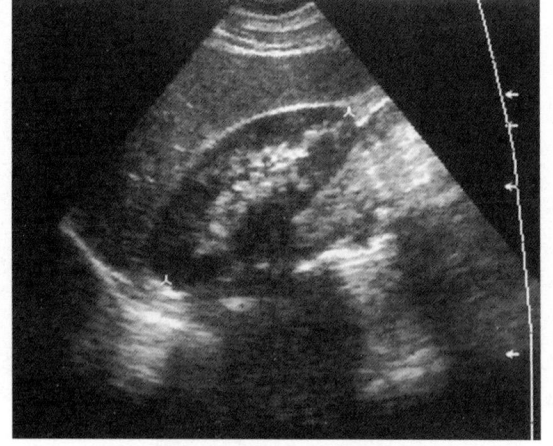

Labeled: **RT KID SAG LONG AXIS**

4. Same image as number 3 *without measurement calipers.*

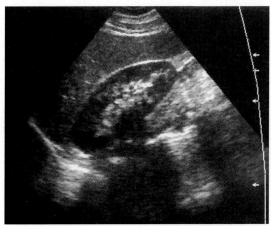

Labeled: **RT KID SAG LONG AXIS**

SCANNING TIP: If the superior and inferior poles were adequately demonstrated on the long axis images, numbers 5 and/or 6 may be omitted.

PART III

5. Longitudinal image of the right kidney superior pole.

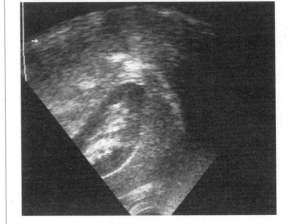

Labeled: RT KID SAG SUP POLE

6. Longitudinal image of the right kidney inferior pole.

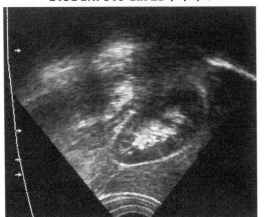

Labeled: RT KID SAG INF POLE

7. Longitudinal image of the right kidney just medial to the long axis.

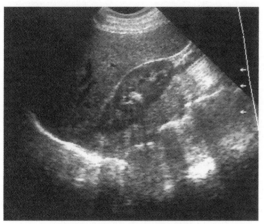

Labeled: **RT KID SAG MED**

8. Longitudinal image of the right kidney just lateral to the long axis to include part of the liver for parenchyma comparison.

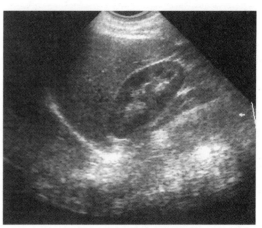

Labeled: **RT KID SAG LAT**

PART III

Right Kidney • Axial Images

9. Axial image of the right kidney superior pole.

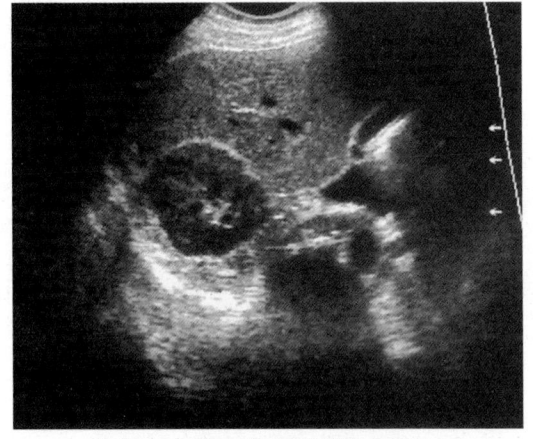

Labeled: **RT KID TRV SUP POLE**

10. Axial image of the right kidney midportion to include the hilum and *anterior to posterior measurement.*

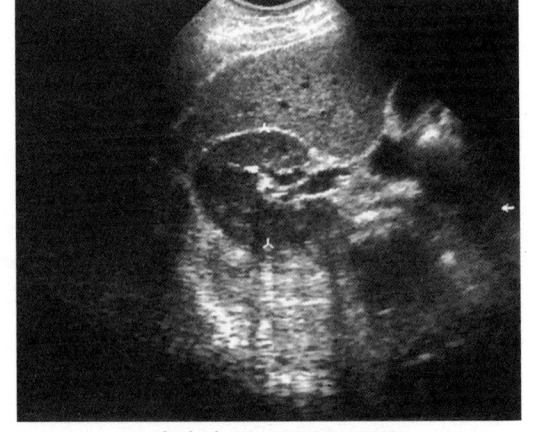

Labeled: **RT KID TRV MID**

11. Same image as number 10 *without measurement calipers.*

12. Axial image of the right kidney inferior pole.

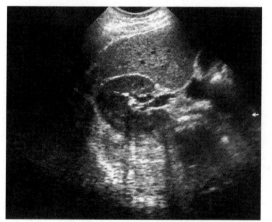

Labeled: **RT KID TRV MID**

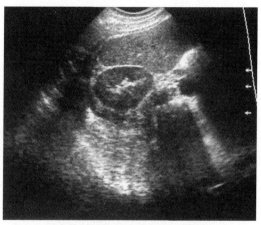

Labeled: **RT KID TRV INF POLE**

Left Kidney • Longitudinal Images

13. Long axis image of the left kidney *with superior to inferior measurement.*

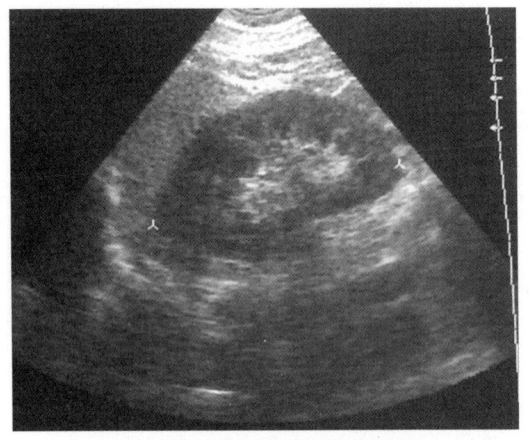

Labeled: **LT KID COR LONG AXIS**

14. Same image as number 13 *without measurement calipers.*

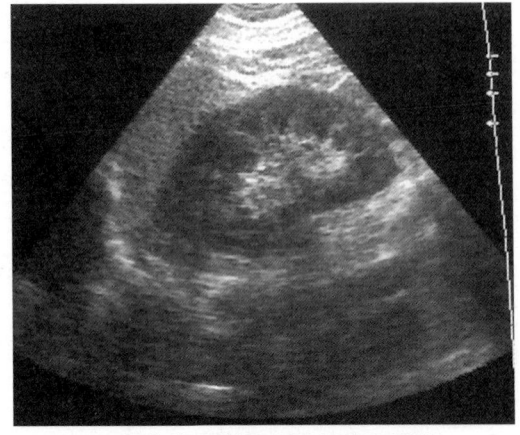

Labeled: **LT KID COR LONG AXIS**

15. Long axis image of the left kidney *with superior to inferior measurement.*

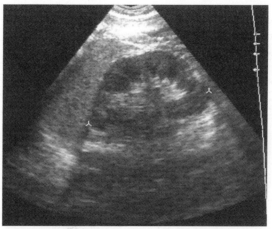

Labeled: **LT KID COR LONG AXIS**

16. Same image as number 15 *without measurement calipers.*

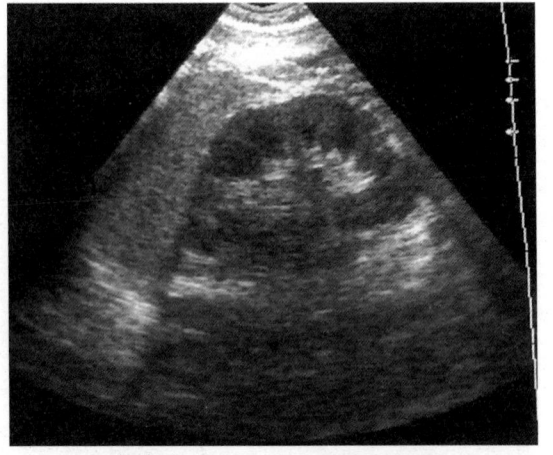

Labeled: **LT KID COR LONG AXIS**

SCANNING TIP: If the superior and inferior poles were adequately demonstrated on the long axis images, numbers 17 and/or 18 may be omitted.

17. Longitudinal image of the left kidney superior pole with part of the spleen for parenchyma comparison.

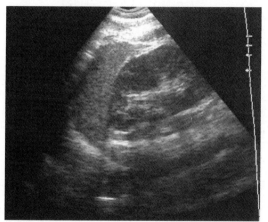

Labeled: **LT KID COR SUP POLE**

18. Longitudinal image of the left kidney inferior pole.

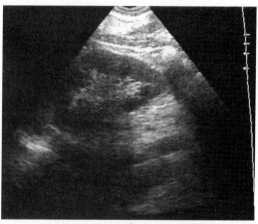

Labeled: **LT KID COR INF POLE**

PART III

19. Longitudinal image of the left kidney just anterior to the long axis.

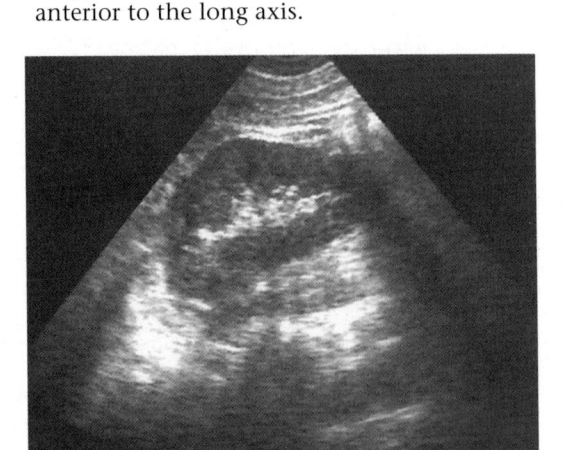

Labeled: **LT KID COR ANT**

20. Longitudinal image of the left kidney just posterior to the long axis.

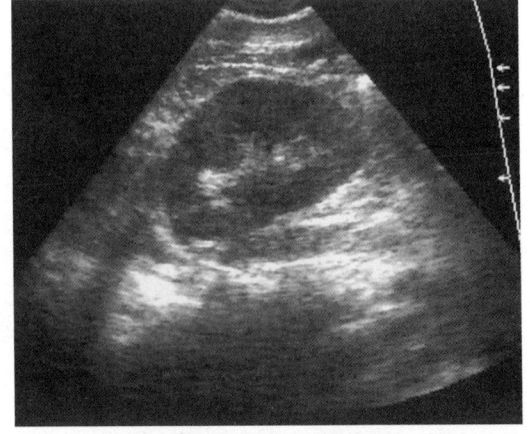

Labeled: **LT KID COR POST**

Left Kidney • Axial Images

21. Axial image of the left kidney superior pole.

22. Axial image of the left kidney midportion to include the hilum and *anterior to posterior measurement.*

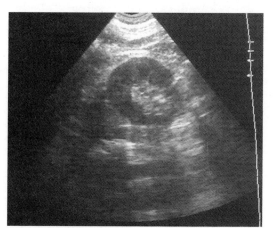

Labeled: **LT KID LT TRV SUP POLE**

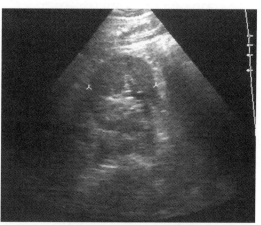

Labeled: **LT KID LT TRV MID**

23. Same image as number 22 *without measurement calipers*.

24. Axial image of the left kidney inferior pole.

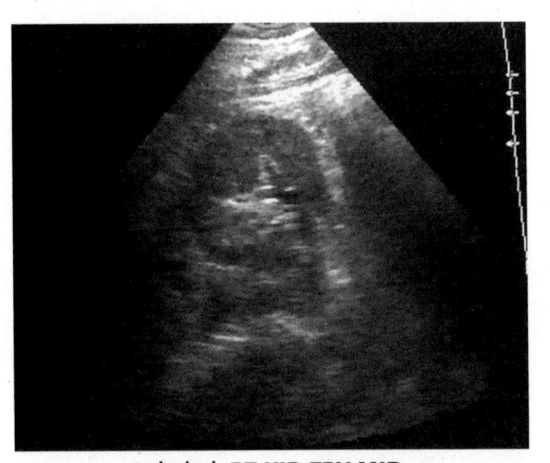

Labeled: **RT KID TRV MID**

Labeled: **LT KID LT TRV INF POLE**

Spleen Study With Limited Abdomen

Spleen • Longitudinal Images

1. Long axis image of the spleen.

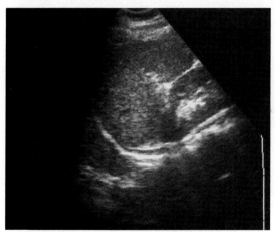

Labeled: **SPLEEN COR LONG AXIS**

SCANNING TIP: If the adjacent pleural space and a portion of the left kidney were adequately demonstrated on number 1, numbers 2 and/or 3 may be omitted.

2. Superior longitudinal image of the spleen to include the adjacent pleural space.

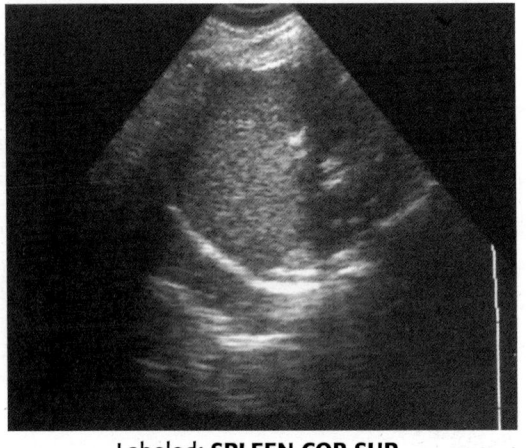

Labeled: **SPLEEN COR SUP**

3. Inferior longitudinal image of the spleen to include part of the left kidney for parenchyma comparison.

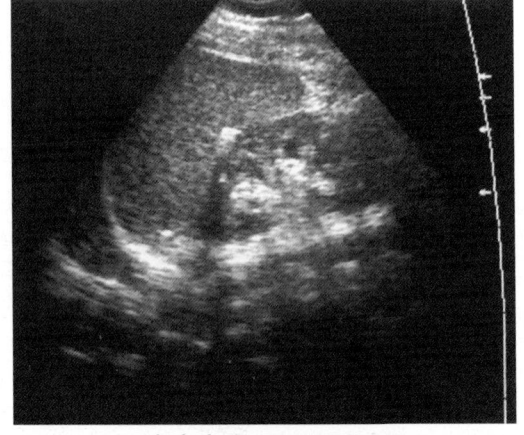

Labeled: **SPLEEN COR INF**

Spleen • Axial Images

4. Axial image of the spleen to include both anterior and posterior margins.

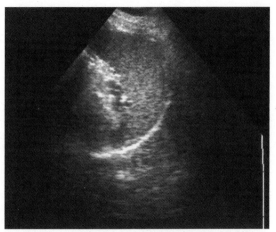

Labeled: **SPLEEN LT TRV**

SCANNING TIP: If the anterior and posterior margins were adequately demonstrated on number 4, numbers 5 and/or 6 may be omitted.

5. Axial image of the spleen to include both anterior margin and splenic hilum.

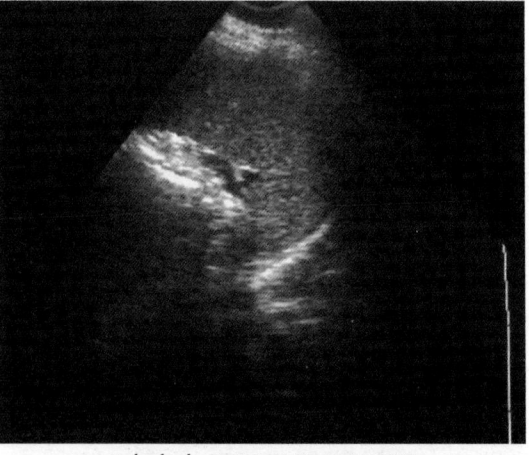

Labeled: **SPLEEN LT TRV ANT**

6. Axial image of the spleen to include the posterior margin.

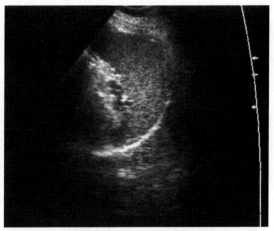

Labeled: **SPLEEN LT TRV POST**

SCANNING TIP: Take an additional image of the superior and/or inferior poles if they are not clearly represented on the long axis image. Label accordingly.

Left Kidney • Longitudinal Image

7. Long axis image of the left kidney.

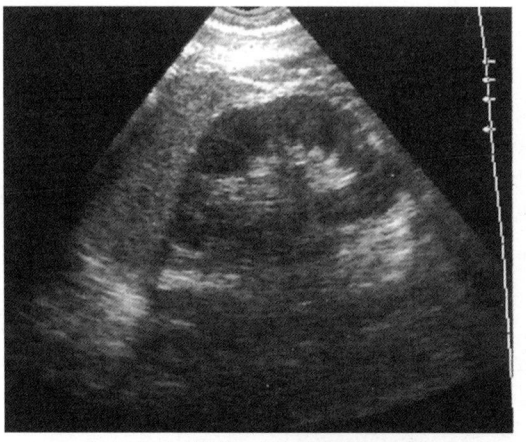

Labeled: **LT KID SAG LONG AXIS**

Left Kidney • Axial Image

8. Axial image of the left kidney midportion to include the hilum.

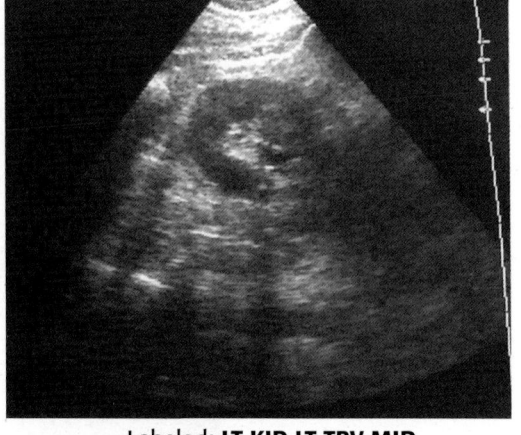

Labeled: **LT KID LT TRV MID**

THE PELVIS

SECTION ONE ▪ Image Protocol for the Transabdominal Sonographic Study of the Female Pelvis

Criteria

- Begin studies with a survey of pelvic structures in at least 2 scanning planes.
  - No single-organ examinations are performed.
  - Do not share study results with the patient. Legally, only a physician can give diagnoses.

Transabdominal Female Pelvis Study

Vagina, Uterus, and Pelvic Cavity • Longitudinal Images

Longitudinal images begin with representative images of the pelvic cavity followed by a long axis image of the uterus.

1. Longitudinal image of the midline of the pelvic cavity just superior to the symphysis pubis.

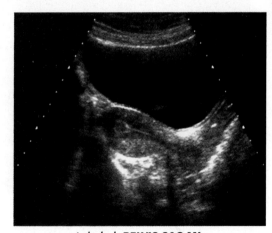

Labeled: **PELVIS SAG ML**

2. Longitudinal image of the right adnexa that may include part of the uterus depending on its position.

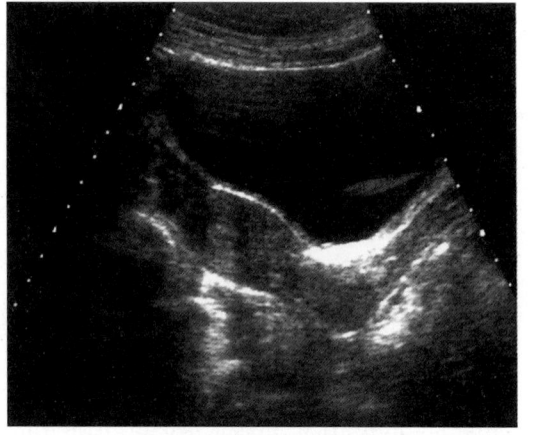

Labeled: **PELVIS SAG R1**

3. Longitudinal image to include the right lateral wall of the bladder and pelvic sidewall.

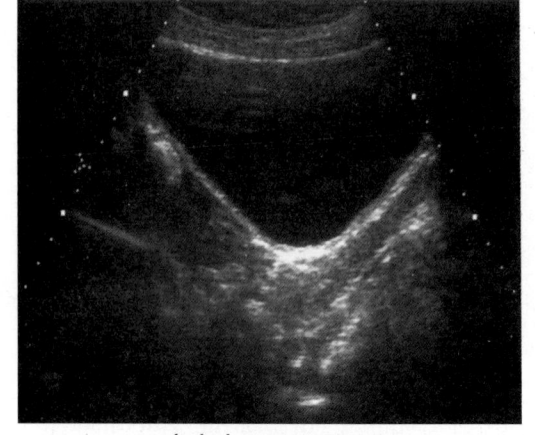

Labeled: **PELVIS SAG R2**

4. Longitudinal image of the left adnexa that may include part of the uterus depending on its position.

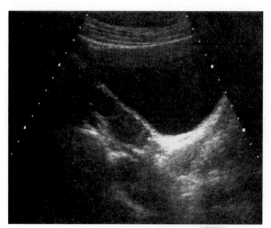

Labeled: **PELVIS SAG L1**

5. Longitudinal image to include the left lateral wall of the bladder and pelvic sidewall.

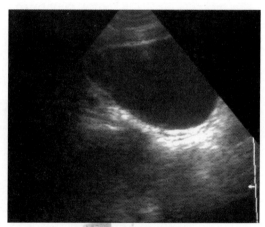

Labeled: **PELVIS SAG L2**

6. Long axis image of the uterus to include as much endometrial cavity as possible *with uterine length (superior to inferior) and height (anterior to posterior) measurements.*

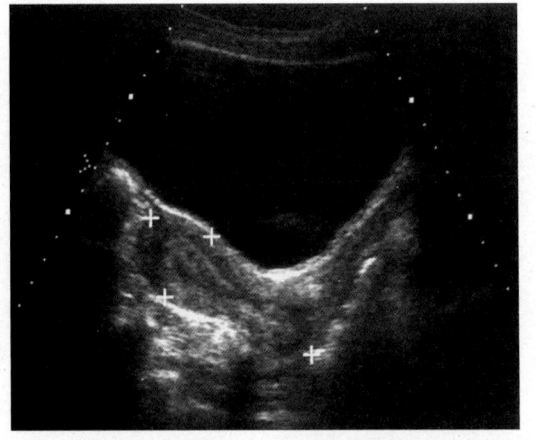

Labeled: **UT SAG LONG AXIS**

7. Same image as number 6 *without calipers.*

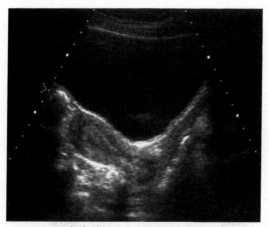

Labeled: **UT SAG LONG AXIS**

SCANNING TIP: It may be necessary to take an additional image demonstrating the long axis of the endometrial, endocervical, and vaginal canals. If so, label the image as follows: **UT SAG**

Vagina, Uterus, and Pelvic Cavity • Axial Images

8. Axial image of the vagina.

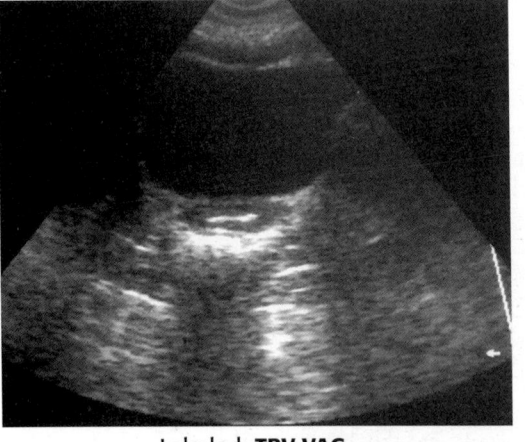

Labeled: **TRV VAG**

9. Axial image of the cervix.

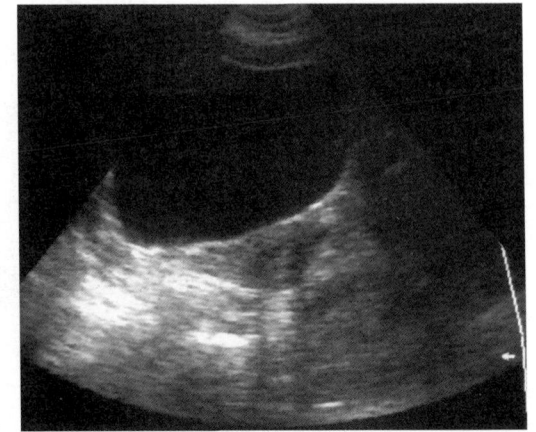

Labeled: **TRV CERX**

10. Axial image of the uterus body.

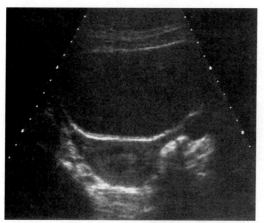

Labeled: **TRV UT BODY**

11. Axial image of the uterus fundus *measuring uterine width (right to left).*

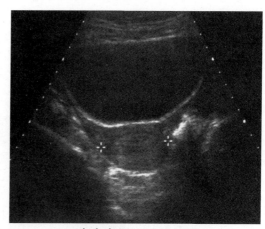

Labeled: **TRV UT FUNDUS**

12. Same image as number 11 *without calipers*.

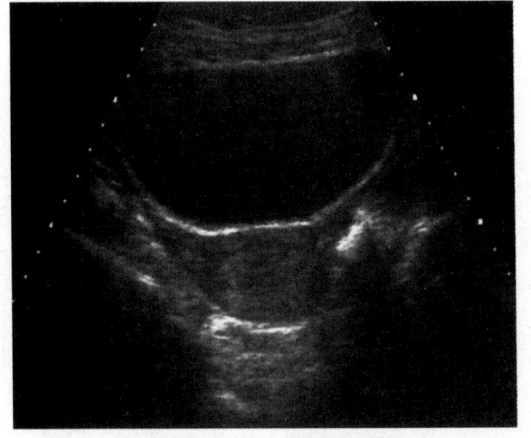

Labeled: **TRV UT FUNDUS**

Right Ovary • Longitudinal Images

13. Long axis image of the right ovary *measuring length (superior to inferior) and height (anterior to posterior).*

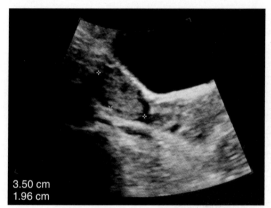

3.50 cm
1.96 cm

Labeled: **RT OV SAG LONG AXIS**
(Courtesy University of Virginia Health Systems
Imaging Center, Charlottesville, Va.)

SCANNING TIP: If this image of the ovary was angled from midline, then the image is obliqued and the image is labeled as follows:
RT OV SAG OBL LONG AXIS

14. Same image as number 13 *without calipers*.

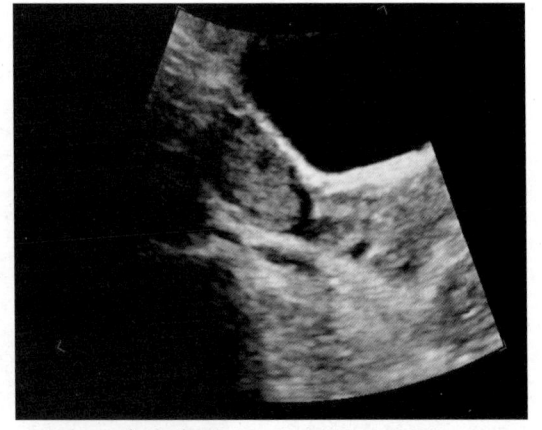

Labeled: **RT OV SAG LONG AXIS**
(Courtesy University of Virginia Health Systems Imaging Center.)

Right Ovary • Axial Images

15. Axial image of the right ovary *with width (right to left) measurement.*

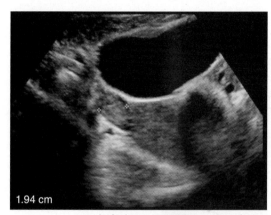

1.94 cm

Labeled: **RT OV TRV**
(Courtesy University of Virginia Health Systems
Imaging Center.)

SCANNING TIP: If this image of the ovary was angled from midline, then the image is obliqued and the image is labeled as follows:
RT OV TRV OBL

16. Same image as number 15 *without calipers*.

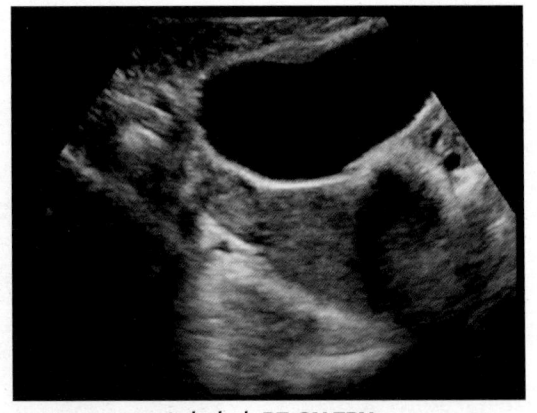

Labeled: **RT OV TRV**
(Courtesy University of Virginia Health Systems Imaging Center.)

Left Ovary • Longitudinal Images

17. Long axis image of the left ovary *measuring length (superior to inferior) and height (anterior to posterior).*

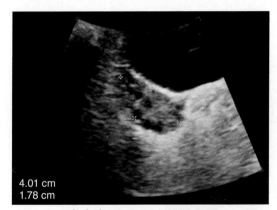

4.01 cm
1.78 cm

Labeled: **LT V SAG LONG AXIS**
(Courtesy University of Virginia Health Systems
Imaging Center.)

SCANNING TIP: If this image of the ovary was angled from midline, then the image is obliqued and the image is labeled as follows:
LT OV SAG OBL LONG AXIS

18. Same image as number 17 *without calipers*.

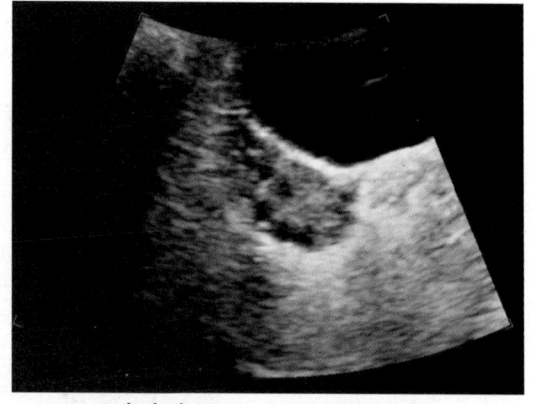

Labeled: **LT OV SAG LONG AXIS**
(Courtesy University of Virginia Health Systems Imaging Center.)

Left Ovary • Axial Images

19. Axial image of the left ovary *with width (right to left) measurement.*

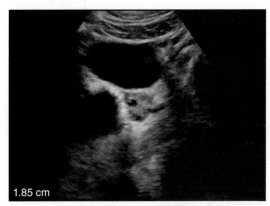

1.85 cm

Labeled: **LT OV TRV**
(Courtesy University of Virginia Health Systems
Imaging Center.)

SCANNING TIP: If this image of the ovary was
angled from midline, then the image is obliqued
and the image is labeled as follows:
RT OV TRV OBL

20. Same image as number 19 *without calipers*.

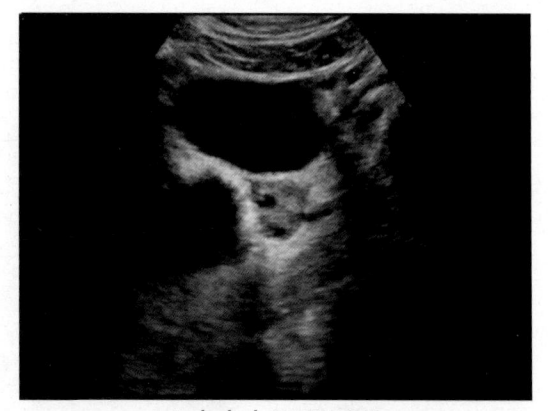

Labeled: **LT OV TRV**
(Courtesy University of Virginia Health Systems Imaging Center.)

SECTION TWO ■ Image Protocol for the Transvaginal Sonographic Study of the Female Pelvis

Criteria

In most cases, "trans" or "endo" vaginal sonography is used in conjunction with transabdominal sonography when pelvic contents require further evaluation.

- Verbal or written consent is required from the patient. Explain the details of the examination; inform the patient that the examination is virtually painless, that the inserted transducer feels like a tampon, and that the examination is necessary for the interpreting physician to make an accurate diagnosis.
- The examination should be chaperoned by a female health care professional. The initials of the witness should be included as part of the film labeling.
- Begin studies with a survey of pelvic structures in at least 2 scanning planes.
- Do not share study results with the patient. Legally, only a physician can give a diagnosis.

Transvaginal Female Pelvis Study

Uterus and Adnexa • Transvaginal Longitudinal Images

1. Longitudinal midline image. If the long axis of the uterus is visualized, then *include length and height measurements.*

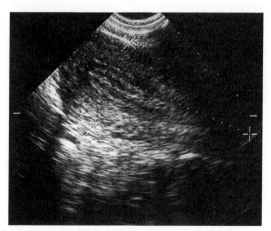

Labeled: **TV SAG ML** or **TV SAG ML UT LONG AXIS** (**"TV"** = transvaginal)

2. Same image as number 1 *without calipers*.

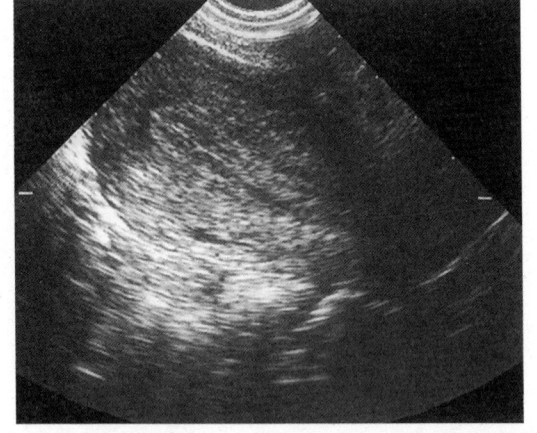

Labeled: **TV SAG ML** or **TV SAG ML UT LONG AXIS**

SCANNING TIP: If the long axis was not visualized at the midline, it should be taken here and label the image as follows:
TV SAG UT LONG AXIS

3. Longitudinal midline image *with anteroposterior measurement* of the endometrium.

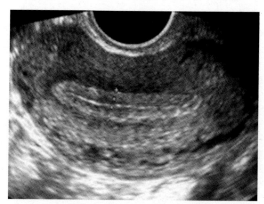

Labeled: **TV SAG ML ENDOM**

SCANNING TIP: The measurement of the endometrium should include anterior and posterior portions of the basal endometrium, the thickest echogenic area, from 1 interface across the endometrial canal to the other interface. The adjacent hypoechoic myometrium and any endometrial fluid should not be part of the measurement.

4. Same image as number 3 *without calipers*.

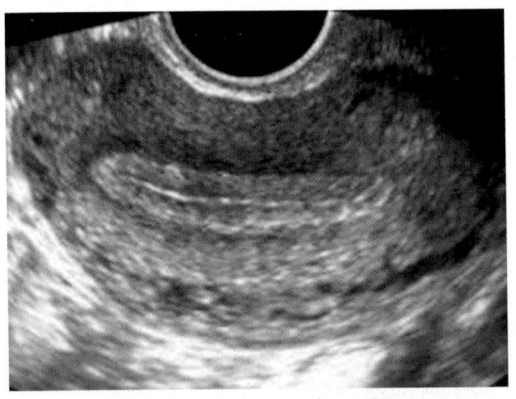

Labeled: **TV SAG ML ENDOM**

5. Longitudinal image of the uterus fundus to include the endometrial cavity.

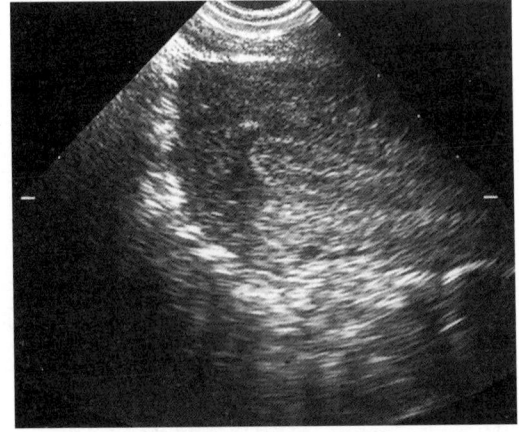

Labeled: **TV SAG FUNDUS**

6. Longitudinal image of the uterus body and cervix to include the endometrial cavity.

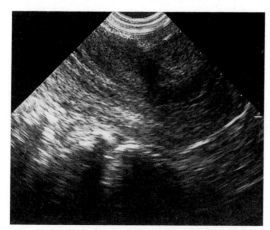

Labeled: **TV SAG BODY CERX**

Uterus and Adnexa • Transvaginal Axial Images

7. Axial image of the uterine fundus *measuring uterine width*.

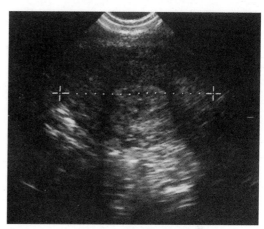

Labeled: **TV COR FUNDUS**

8. Same image as number 7 *without calipers*.

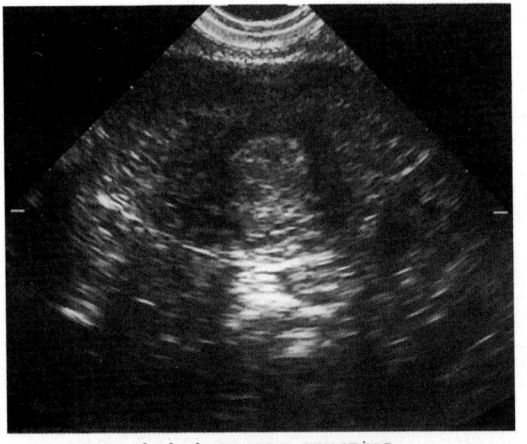

Labeled: **TV COR FUNDUS**

9. Axial image of the uterine body.

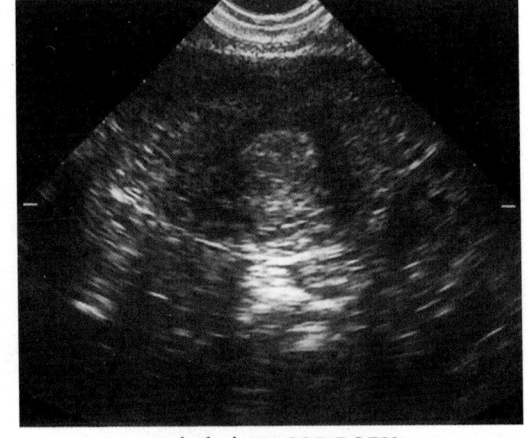

Labeled: **TV COR BODY**

10. Axial image of the cervix.

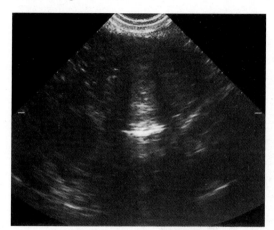

Labeled: **TV COR CERX**

Right Ovary • Transvaginal Axial Images

For the sake of instruction, this assumes that the ovary long axis is visualized in a sagittal plane.

11. Axial image of the right ovary *measuring ovarian width.*

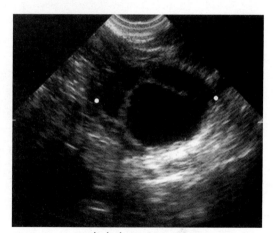

Labeled: **TV COR RT OV**

12. Same image as number 11 *without calipers*.

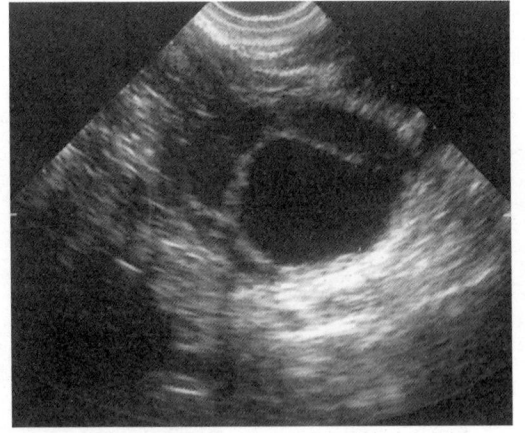

Labeled: **TV COR RT OV**

Right Ovary • Transvaginal Longitudinal Images

For the sake of instruction, this assumes that the ovary long axis is visualized in a sagittal plane.

13. Long axis image of the right ovary *measuring ovarian length and height.*

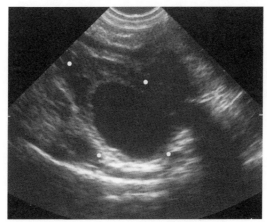

Labeled: **TV SAG RT OV LONG AXIS**

14. Same image as number 13 *without calipers*.

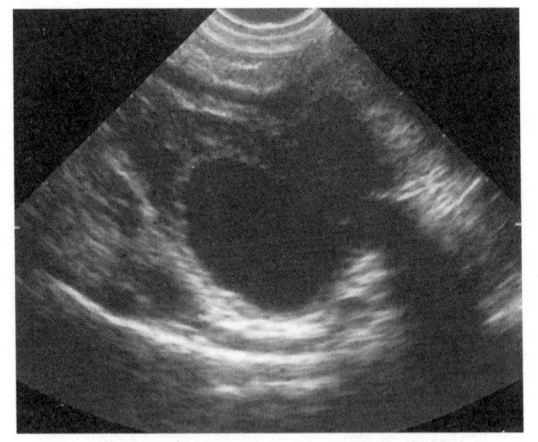

Labeled: **TV SAG RT OV LONG AXIS**

Left Ovary • Transvaginal Axial Images
Coronal Plane • Inferior Approach

For the sake of instruction, this assumes that the ovary long axis is visualized in a sagittal plane.

15. Axial image of the left ovary *measuring ovarian width.*

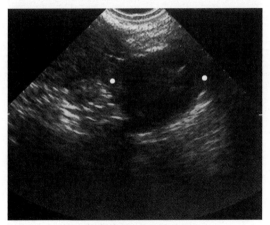

Labeled: **TV COR LT OV**

16. Same image as number 15 *without calipers*.

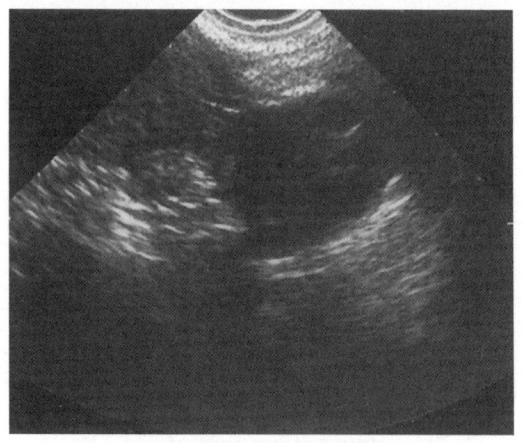

Labeled: **TV COR LT OV**

Left Ovary • Transvaginal Longitudinal Images

For the sake of instruction, this assumes that the ovary long axis is visualized in a sagittal plane.

17. Long axis image of the left ovary *measuring ovarian length and height.*

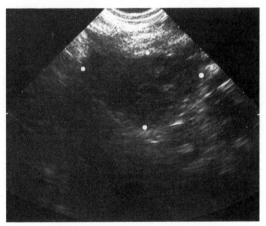

Labeled: **TV SAG LT OV LONG AXIS**

18. Same image as number 17 *without calipers.*

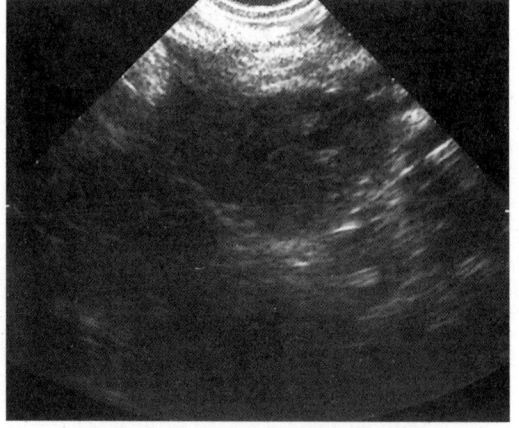

Labeled: **TV SAG LT OV LONG AXIS**

SECTION THREE ▪ Image Protocols for Sonographic Studies of the Male Pelvis

- Transrectal Prostate Gland Study*
- Scrotum Study
- Penis Study

---

*Images in this section are courtesy the Ultrasound Department of Methodist Hospital, Houston, Tex.

Criteria

- These examinations should be witnessed by another health care professional, whose initials should be part of the film labeling. For transrectal or endorectal prostate evaluations, the patient's verbal or written consent is also required.
- Begin studies with a survey of pelvic structures in at least 2 scanning planes.
- Do not share study results with the patient. Legally, only physicians can give a diagnosis.

Transrectal Prostate Gland Study

SCANNING TIP: The required images are a small representation of what a sonographer visualizes during a study. Therefore, the images should provide the interpreting physician with the most telling and technically accurate information available.

Prostate • Axial Images

1. Axial image of the seminal vesicles.

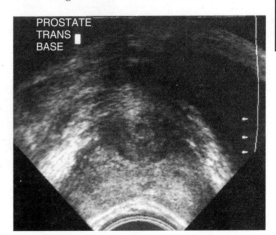

Labeled: **ER TRV SEM V ("ER" indicates endorectal)**

SCANNING TIP: Because of the limited field of view, both seminal vesicles may not be entirely visible on a single view. If so, take these additional images:

2. Axial image of the right seminal vesicle to include its right lateral margin.

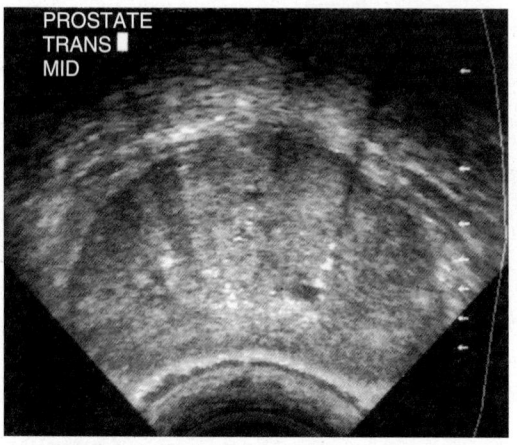

Labeled: **ER TRV SEM V RT**

3. Axial image of the left seminal vesicle to include its left lateral margin.

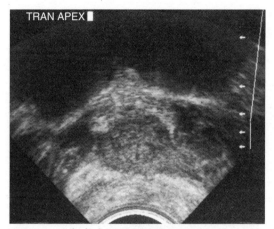

Labeled: **ER TRV SEM V LT**

4. Axial image of the base of the prostate.

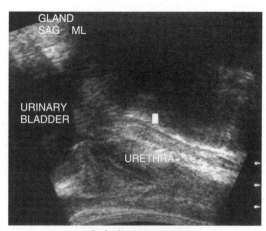

Labeled: **ER TRV BASE**

5. Axial image of the midprostate.

6. Axial image of the apex of the prostate.

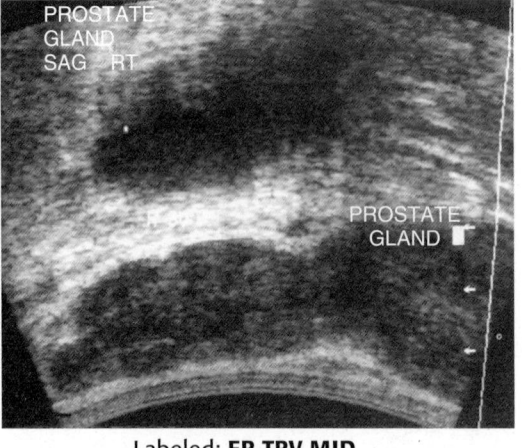

Labeled: **ER TRV MID**

Labeled: **ER TRV APEX**

Prostate • Longitudinal Images

7. Longitudinal midline image of the prostate.

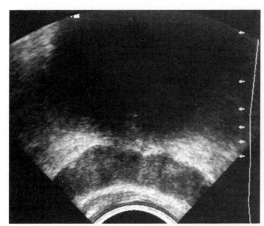

Labeled: **ER SAG ML**

8. Longitudinal image of the right lateral portion of the prostate gland and seminal vesicle.

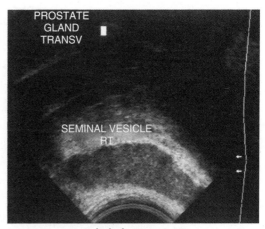

Labeled: **ER SAG RT**

9. Longitudinal image of the left lateral portion of the prostate gland and seminal vesicle.

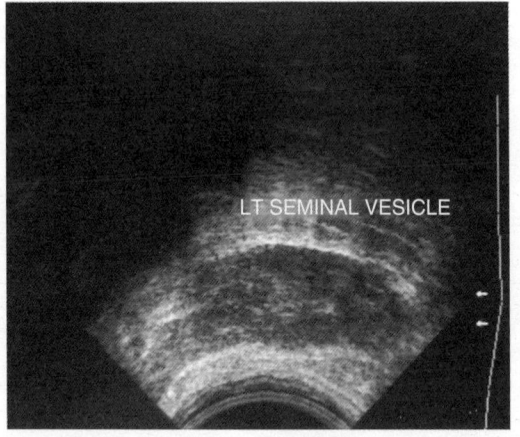

LT SEMINAL VESICLE

Labeled: **ER SAG LT**

SCANNING TIP: The required images are a small representation of what a sonographer visualizes during a study. Therefore, the images should provide the interpreting physician with the most telling and technically accurate information available.

Scrotum • Right Hemiscrotum • Longitudinal Images

1. Long axis image of the spermatic cord at normal respiration or rest with *anterior to posterior measurement.*

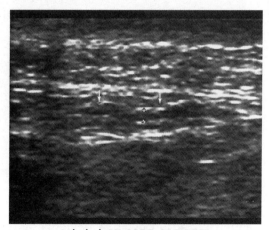

Labeled: **RT CORD SAG REST**

2. Same image as number 1 *without calipers.*

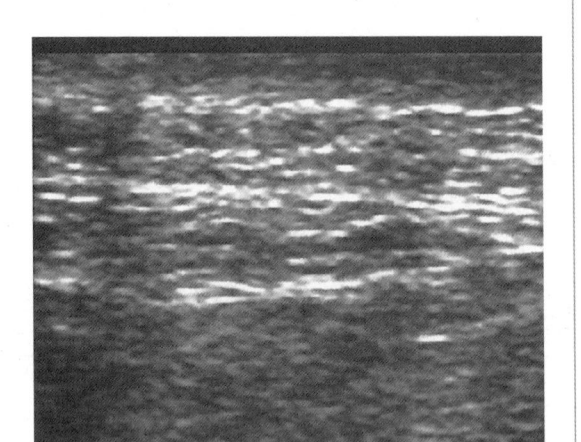

Labeled: **RT CORD SAG REST**

3. Long axis image of the spermatic cord during the Valsalva maneuver *with anterior to posterior measurement.*

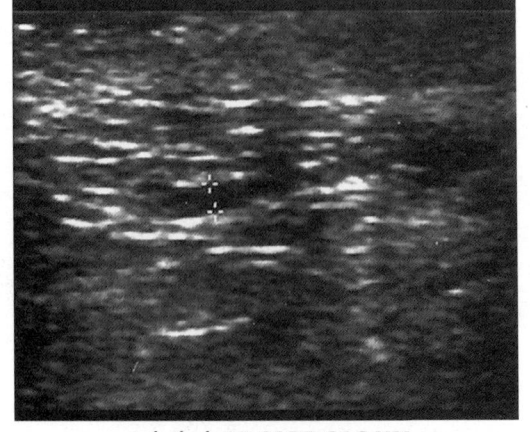

Labeled: **RT CORD SAG VAL**

4. Same image as number 3 *without calipers*.

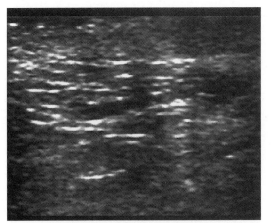

Labeled: **RT CORD SAG VAL**

5. Longitudinal image of the head of the epididymis.

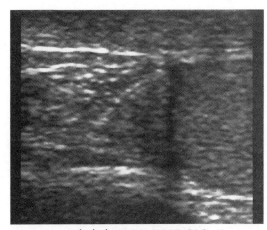

Labeled: **RT EPI HEAD SAG**

6. Longitudinal image of the right testis at its most superior margin.

Labeled: **RT TESTIS SAG SUP**

7. Longitudinal image of the midportion of the right testis.

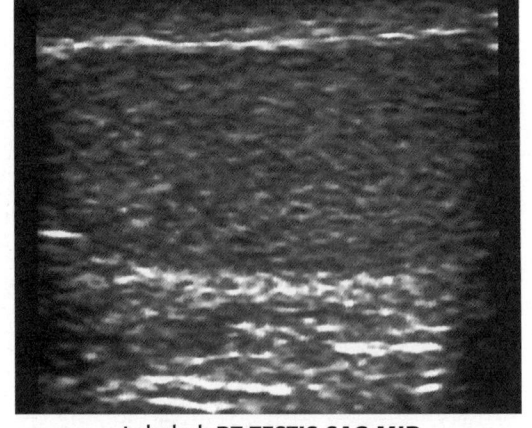

Labeled: **RT TESTIS SAG MID**

8. Long axis image of the spermatic right testis *with superior to inferior measurement.*

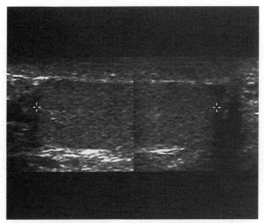

Labeled: **RT TESTIS SAG LONG AXIS**

SCANNING TIP: If necessary, use dual imaging to obtain the entire long axis of the testis on the image.

9. Same image as number 8 *without calipers*.

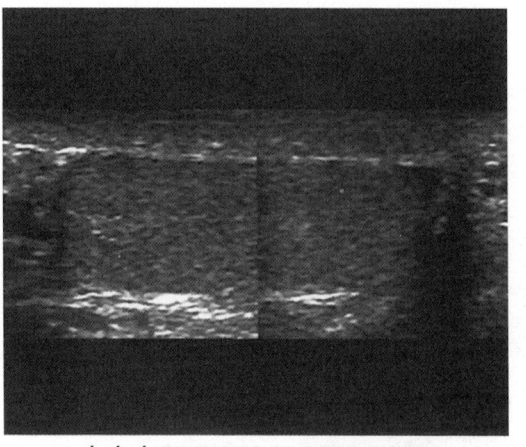

Labeled: **RT TESTIS SAG LONG AXIS**

10. Longitudinal image of the medial portion of the right testis.

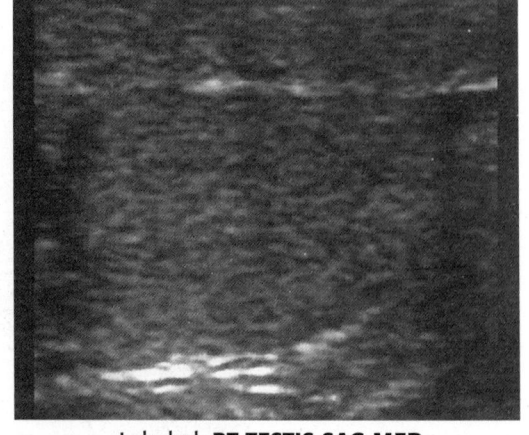

Labeled: **RT TESTIS SAG MED**

11. Longitudinal image of the lateral portion of the right testis.

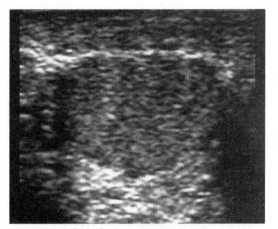

Labeled: **RT TESTIS SAG LAT**

12. Longitudinal image of the right testis at its most inferior margin.

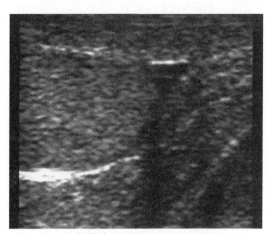

Labeled: **RT TESTIS SAG INF**

13. Longitudinal image of the tail of the epididymis (if visualized).

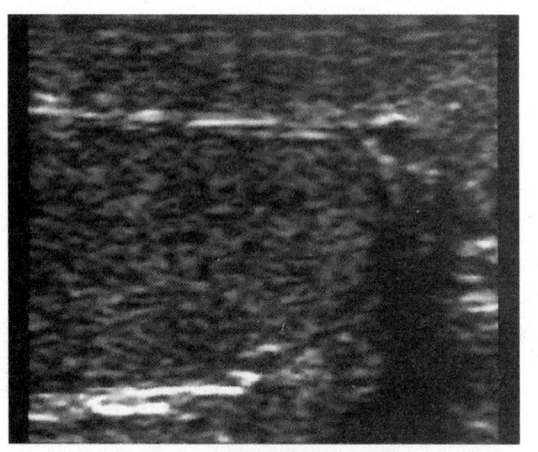

Labeled: **RT EPI TAIL SAG**

Scrotum • Right Hemiscrotum • Axial Images

14. Axial image of the spermatic cord at normal respiration or rest *with anterior to posterior measurement.*

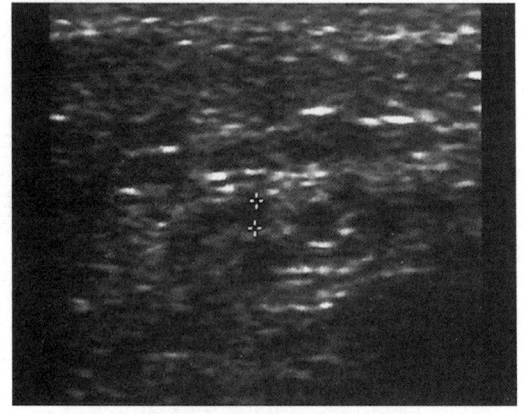

Labeled: **RT CORD TRV REST**

15. Same image as number 14 *without calipers.*

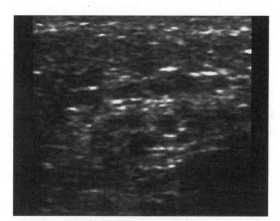

Labeled: **RT CORD TRV REST**

16. Axial image of the spermatic cord during the Valsalva maneuver *with anterior to posterior measurement.*

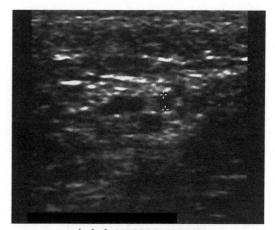

Labeled: **RT CORD TRV VAL**

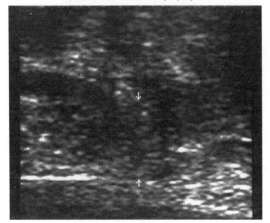

18. Axial image of the epididymal head.

Labeled: **RT EPI HEAD TRV**

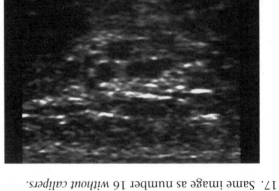

17. *Same image as number 16 without calipers.*

Labeled: **RT CORD TRV VAL**

19. Axial image of the superior portion of the right testis.

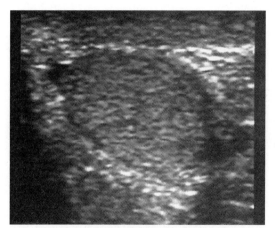

Labeled: **RT TESTIS TRV SUP**

20. Axial image of the midportion of the right testis *with medial to lateral measurement.*

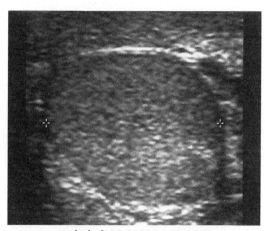

Labeled: **RT TESTIS TRV MID**

Labeled: RT TESTIS TRV MID

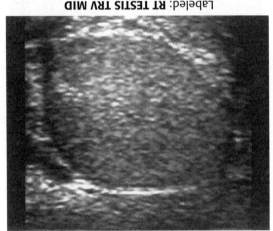

21. Same image as number 20 without calipers.

Labeled: RT TESTIS TRV INF

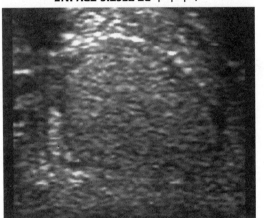

22. Axial image of the inferior portion of the right testis.

23. Axial image of the tail of the epididymis (if visualized).

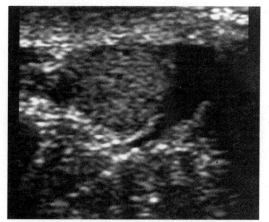

Labeled: **RT TESTIS TRV INF/EPI TAIL**

Scrotum • Left Hemiscrotum • Longitudinal Images

1. Long axis image of the spermatic cord at normal respiration or rest *with anterior to posterior measurement.*

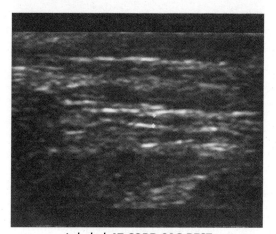

Labeled: **LT CORD SAG REST**

2. Same image as number 1 without calipers.

Labeled: LT CORD SAG REST

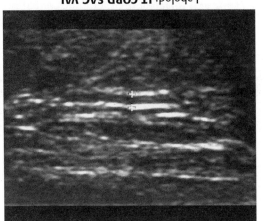

3. Long axis image of the spermatic cord during the Valsalva maneuver with anterior to posterior measurement.

Labeled: LT CORD SAG VAL

4. Same image as number 3 *without calipers*.

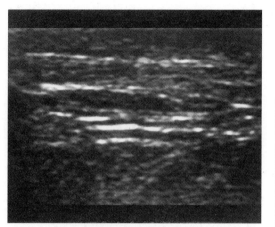

Labeled: **LT CORD SAG VAL**

5. Longitudinal image of the head of the epididymis.

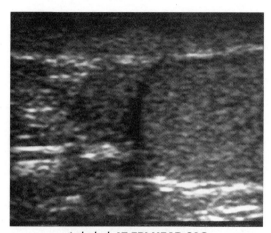

Labeled: **LT EPI HEAD SAG**

6. Longitudinal image of the left testis at its most superior margin.

Labeled: **LT TESTIS SAG SUP**

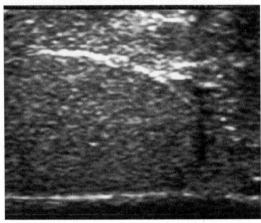

7. Longitudinal image of the midportion of the left testis.

Labeled: **LT TESTIS SAG MID**

8. Long axis image of the left testis with *superior to inferior measurement.*

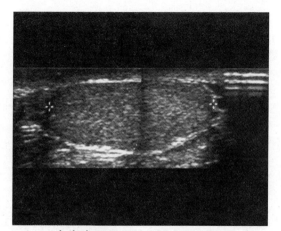

Labeled: **LT TESTIS SAG LONG AXIS**

SCANNING TIP: If necessary, use dual imaging to obtain the entire long axis of the testis on the image.

9. Same image as number 8 *without calipers*.

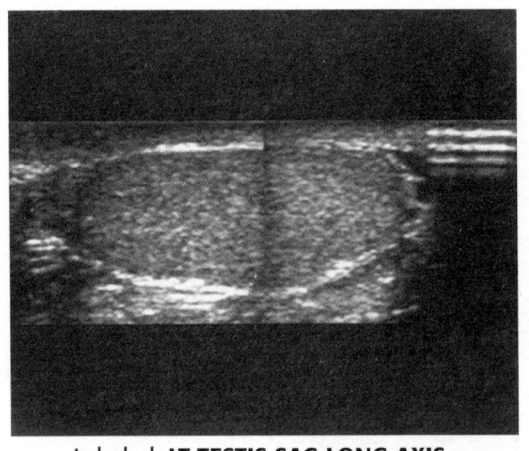

Labeled: **LT TESTIS SAG LONG AXIS**

10. Longitudinal image of the medial portion of the left testis.

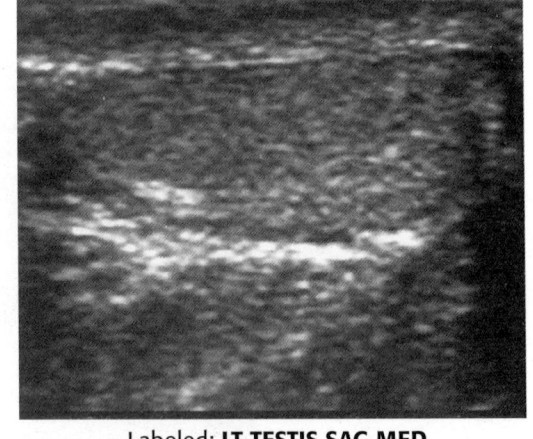

Labeled: **LT TESTIS SAG MED**

11. Longitudinal image of the lateral portion of the left testis.

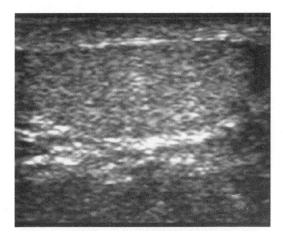

Labeled: **LT TESTIS SAG LAT**

12. Longitudinal image of the left testis at its most inferior margin.

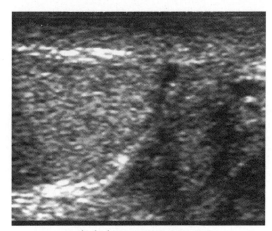

Labeled: **LT TESTIS SAG INF**

13. Longitudinal image of the tail of the epididymis (if visualized).

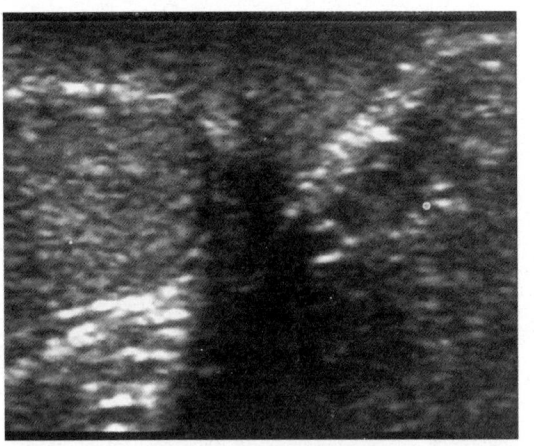

Labeled: **LT EPI TAIL SAG**

Scrotum • Left Hemiscrotum • Axial Images

14. Axial image of the spermatic cord at normal respiration or rest *with anterior to posterior measurement.*

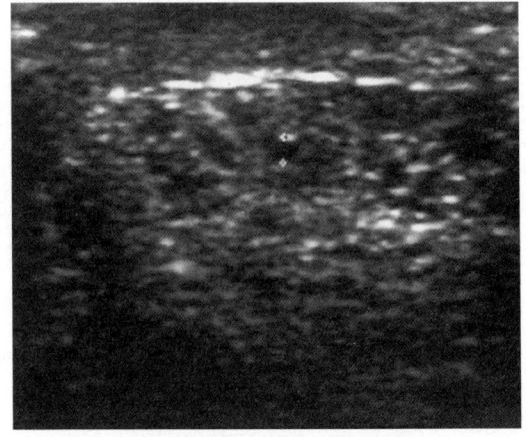

Labeled: **LT CORD TRV REST**

15. Same image as number 14 *without calipers.*

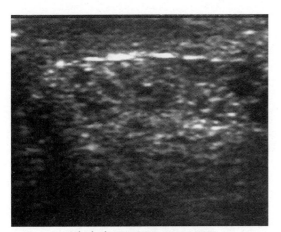

Labeled: **LT CORD TRV REST**

16. Axial image of the spermatic cord during the Valsalva maneuver *with anterior to posterior measurement.*

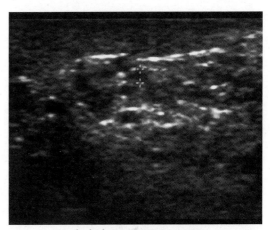

Labeled: **LT CORD TRV VAL**

Labeled: **LT CORD TRV VAL**

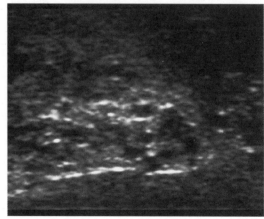

17. Same image as number 16 *without calipers.*

Labeled: **LT EPI HEAD TRV**

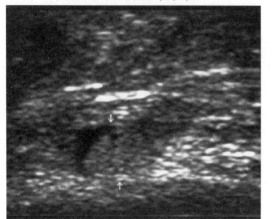

18. Axial image of the epididymal head.

19. Axial image of the superior portion of the left testis.

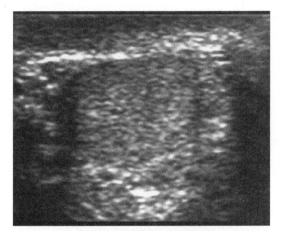

Labeled: **LT TESTIS TRV SUP**

20. Axial image of the midportion of the left testis *with medial to lateral measurement.*

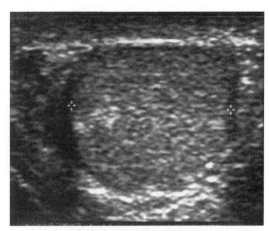

Labeled: **LT TESTIS TRV MID**

21. *Same image as number 20 without calipers.*

Labeled: **LT TESTIS TRV MID**

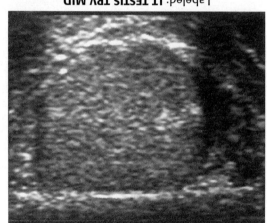

Labeled: **LT TESTIS TRV INF**

22. Axial image of the inferior portion of the left testis.

23. Axial image of the tail of the epididymis (if visualized).

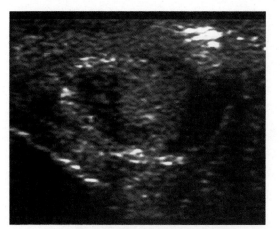

Labeled: **LT TESTIS TRV INF/EPI TAIL**

24. Axial image of the midportion of both testes.

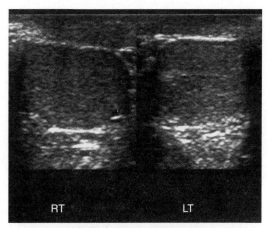

Labeled: **BILAT TESTES TRV**

Penis Study

1. Longitudinal section of the penis.

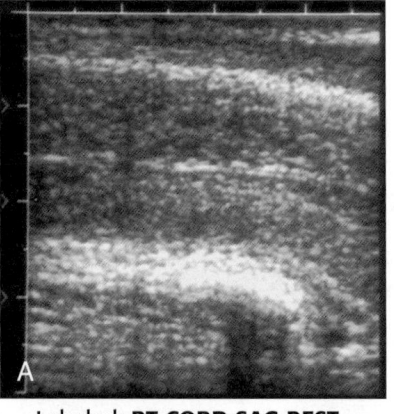

Labeled: **RT CORD SAG REST**

2. Axial section of the penis.

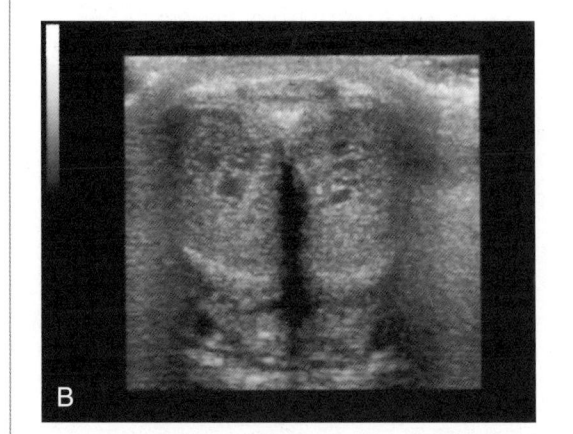

Penis • Longitudinal Images

1. Longitudinal image of the left lateral, superior portion of the penis to include the corpus spongiosum, corpus cavernosum, and cavernosal artery.

   Labeled: **SAG PENIS LT SUP**

2. Longitudinal image of the left lateral, midportion of the penis to include the corpus spongiosum, corpus cavernosum, and cavernosal artery.

   Labeled: **SAG PENIS LT MID**

3. Longitudinal image of the left lateral, inferior portion of the penis to include the corpus spongiosum, corpus cavernosum, and cavernosal artery.

   Labeled: **SAG PENIS LT INF**

4. Longitudinal image of the left lateral glans penis.

   Labeled: **SAG PENIS LT GLANS**

5. Longitudinal image of the right lateral, superior portion of the penis to include the corpus spongiosum, corpus cavernosum, and cavernosal artery.

   Labeled: **SAG PENIS RT SUP**

6. Longitudinal image of the right lateral, midportion of the penis to include the corpus spongiosum, corpus cavernosum, and cavernosal artery.

   Labeled: **SAG PENIS RT MID**

7. Longitudinal image of the right lateral, inferior portion of the penis to include the corpus spongiosum, corpus cavernosum, and cavernosal artery.

   Labeled: **SAG PENIS RT INF**

8. Longitudinal image of the right lateral glans penis.

   Labeled: **SAG PENIS RT GLANS**

Penis • Axial Images

9. Axial image of the superior portion of the penis to include the corpus spongiosum, corpus cavernosum, and cavernosal arteries.

   Labeled: **TRV PENIS SUP**

10. Axial image of the midportion of the penis to include the corpus spongiosum, corpus cavernosum, and cavernosal arteries.

    Labeled: **TRV PENIS MID**

11. Axial image of the inferior portion of the penis to include the corpus spongiosum, corpus cavernosum, and cavernosal arteries.

    Labeled: **TRV PENIS INF**

12. Axial image of the glans penis.

    Labeled: **TRV PENIS GLANS**

OBSTETRICS

SECTION ONE ▪ Image Protocol for the Sonographic Study of the Early First Trimester

Criteria

- No limited studies.
- Before the examination, a patient history including the date of the first day of the patient's last period, gravidity, parity, and history of any pelvic surgery should be taken.
- Begin early first trimester studies with a survey of the uterus and adnexa followed by the pregnancy if present.
- When transvaginal sonography is used in conjunction with the routine transabdominal study, the patient's verbal or written consent is required. Also, the examination should be chaperoned by a female health care professional, whose initials should be included as part of the film labeling.
- Do not share study results with the patient. Legally, only physicians can give a diagnosis.

Early First Trimester Study

SCANNING TIP: Depending on how early the gestation is, it may be helpful to magnify the field of view for the gestational sac images.

Uterus Long Axis

1. Long axis image of the uterus showing the location of the gestational sac.

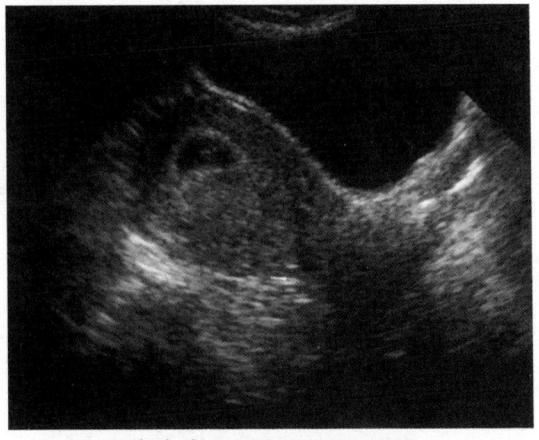

Labeled: **UT SAG LONG AXIS**

Gestational Sac

2. Longitudinal image of the gestational sac *with length (superior to inferior) and depth (anterior to posterior) measurements (calipers inside wall to inside wall).*

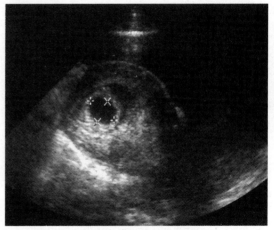

Labeled: **GS SAG OR TRV**

PART V

3. Same image as number 2 *without calipers.*

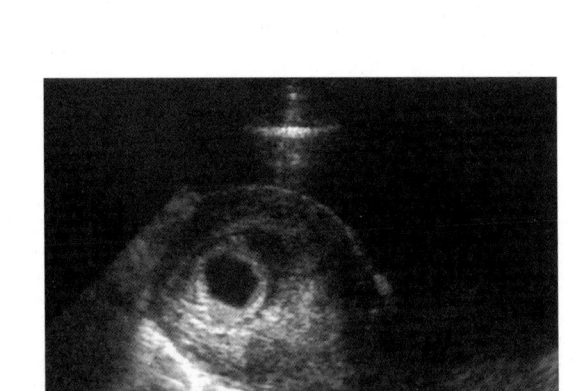

Labeled: **GS SAG OR TRV**

4. Axial image of the gestational sac *with greatest width (right to left) measurement (calipers inside wall to inside wall).*

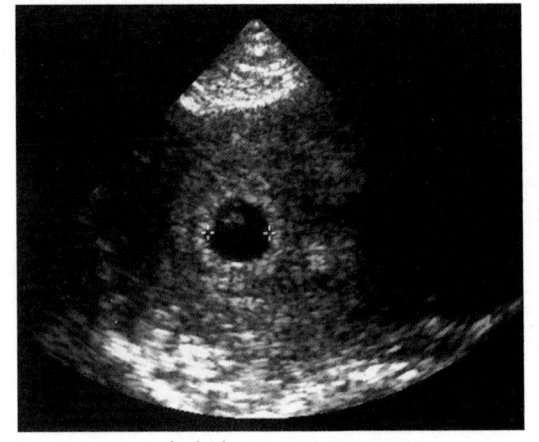

Labeled: **GS SAG OR TRV**

5. Same image as number 4 *without calipers*.

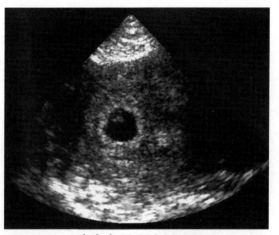

Labeled: **GS SAG OR TRV**

SCANNING TIP: If the yolk sac and/or embryo are present and have not been clearly demonstrated with the gestational sac measurement images, an additional image of the yolk sac and/or embryo should be taken and labeled accordingly.

Yolk Sac and/or Embryo

6. Image demonstrating the yolk sac and/or embryo.

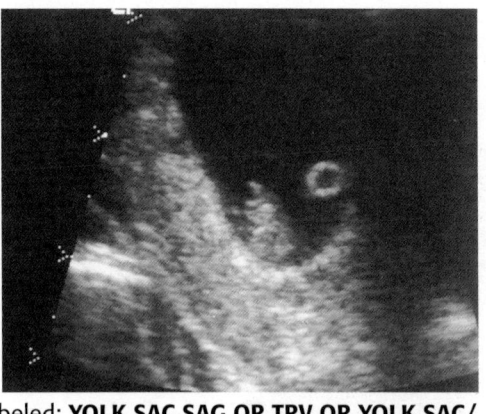

Labeled: **YOLK SAC SAG OR TRV OR YOLK SAC/ EMBRYO SAG OR TRV**

7. Long axis image of embryo *with length (superior to inferior) or crown rump length (CRL) measurement.*

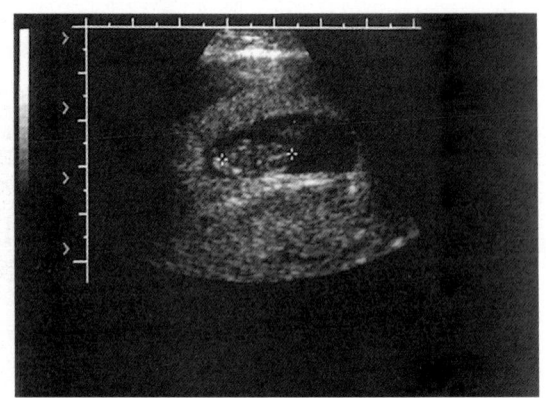

Labeled: **CRL**

8. Same image as number 7 *without calipers*.

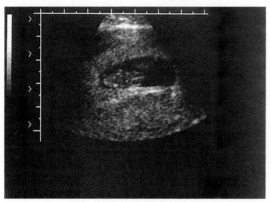

Labeled: **CRL**

9. Doppler documentation of viability.

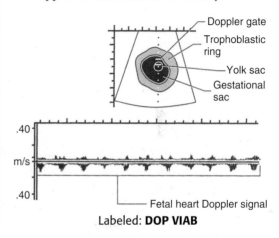

Labeled: **DOP VIAB**

SECTION TWO ▪ Image Protocol for the Sonographic Study of the Late First Trimester

Criteria

- No limited studies.
- Before the examination, a patient history including the date of the first day of the patient's last period, gravidity, parity, and history of any pelvic surgery should be taken.
- Begin late first trimester studies with a survey of the uterus and adnexa followed by the pregnancy if present.
- When transvaginal sonography is used in conjunction with the routine transabdominal study, the patient's verbal or written consent is required. Also, the examination should be chaperoned by a female health care professional, whose initials should be included as part of the film labeling.
- Do not share study results with the patient. Legally, only physicians can give a diagnosis.

Late First Trimester Study

Uterus Long Axis

1. Long axis image of the uterus showing the location of the gestational sac.

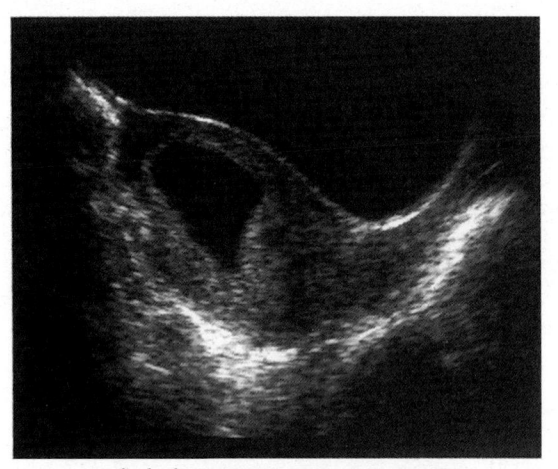

Labeled: **UTERUS SAG LONG AXIS**

SCANNING TIP: Assuming an embryo is identified, the CRL measurement is taken in the scanning plane where its long axis appears.

Gestational Sac

2. Longitudinal image of the gestational sac to include the embryo (if visualized) *with measurement from crown to rump* (if applicable) *and placenta location* (if distinguishable).

3. Axial image of the gestational sac to include the embryo (if visualized) *with measurement from crown to rump* (if applicable) *and placenta location* (if distinguishable).

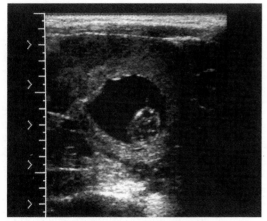

Labeled: **GS SAG or TRV**

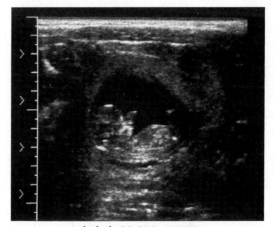

Labeled: **GS SAG or TRV**

4. Same image as number 3 *without calipers* (if applicable).

> **SCANNING TIP:** In this case, the CRL measurement was not applied to the previous image; therefore an additional image demonstrating the longest axis of the embryo with CRL measurement must be taken.

5. Long axis image of the embryo *with measurement from crown to rump.*

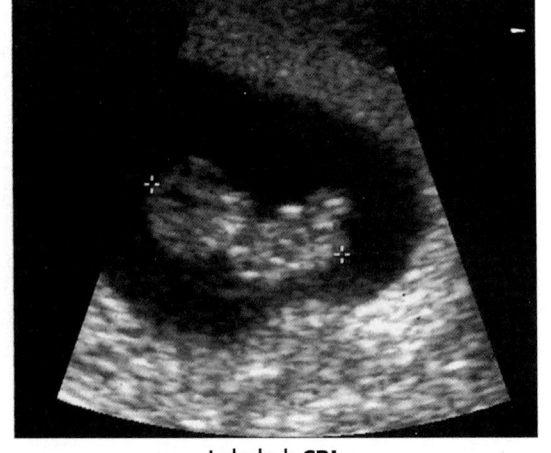

Labeled: **CRL**

6. Same image as number 5 *without calipers.*

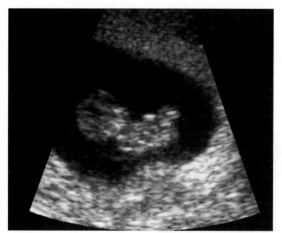

Labeled: **CRL**

SCANNING TIP: In addition to the CRL measurement, some institutions require biparietal diameter, abdominal circumference, and femur length measurements of the embryo during the later part of the first trimester. However, many experts believe that these additional measurements are not necessary because they do not add any new information to the study and they are not as accurate as the CRL measurement for determining gestational age.

7. Optional view(s) of the embryo demonstrating limbs.

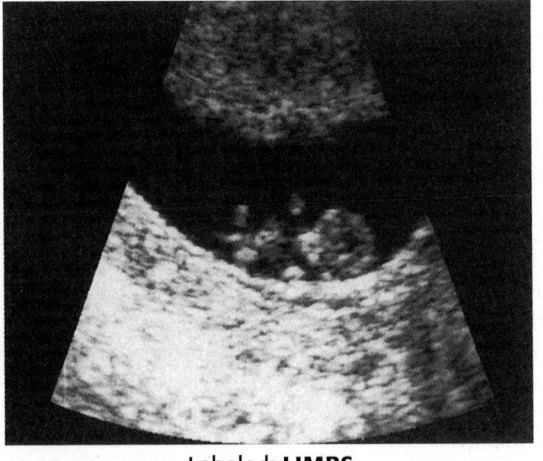

Labeled: **LIMBS**

SCANNING TIP: It may be helpful to magnify the field of view for the limb image(s).

SECTION THREE ▪ Image Protocol for the Sonographic Study of the Second and Third Trimesters

Criteria

- No limited studies.
- Before the examination, a patient history including the date of the first day of the patient's last period, gravidity, parity, and history of any pelvic surgery should be taken.
- Begin late first trimester studies with a survey of the uterus and adnexa followed by the pregnancy if present.
- When transvaginal sonography is used in conjunction with the routine transabdominal study, the patient's verbal or written consent is required. Also, the examination should be chaperoned by a female health care professional, whose initials should be included as part of the film labeling.
- Do not share study results with the patient. Legally, only physicians can give a diagnosis.

Second and Third Trimesters Study

Uterus Long Axis

1. When the trimester allows, obtain long axis image of the uterus and contents or best overall longitudinal representation.

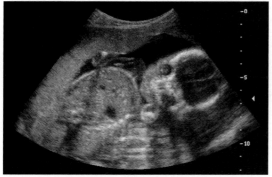

Labeled: **UTERUS SAG**

SCANNING TIP: In this case the trimester was too advanced to image the entire uterus on a single view.

Placenta

2. Longitudinal image of the placenta.

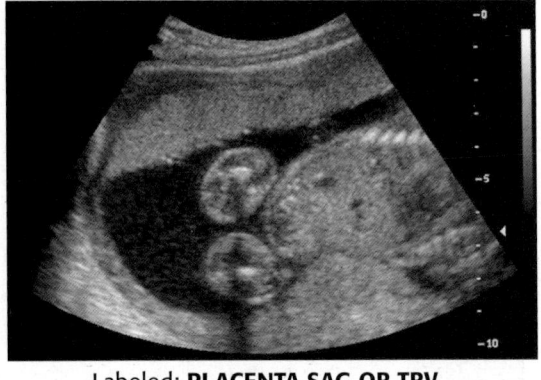

Labeled: **PLACENTA SAG OR TRV**

3. Axial image of the placenta.

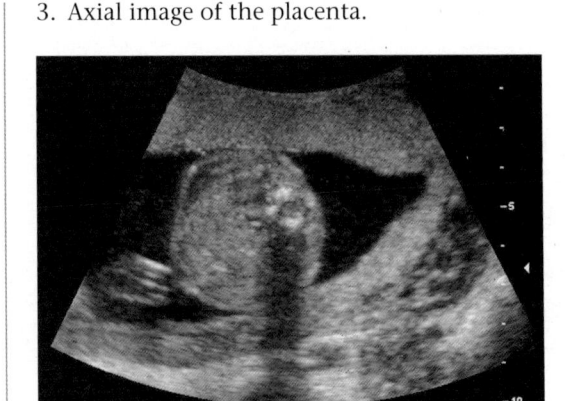

Labeled: **PLACENTA SAG OR TRV**

Cervix

4. Longitudinal image of the cervix to include the internal os.

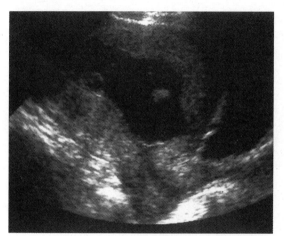

Labeled: **CERVIX SAG**

SCANNING TIP: An image of the lower uterine segment to include the internal os is required to rule out placental previa and to document the cervix. In cases where the head of the fetus or the mother's body habitus inhibit imaging of the lower uterine segment, either an endovaginal or a translabial image must be obtained. The translabial image is obtained with an empty or nearly empty bladder. The transducer is covered with a sheath, condom, or glove and placed between the labia. The transducer is angled so that the cervix is nearly perpendicular to the ultrasound beam.

Longitudinal translabial image of the lower uterine segment.

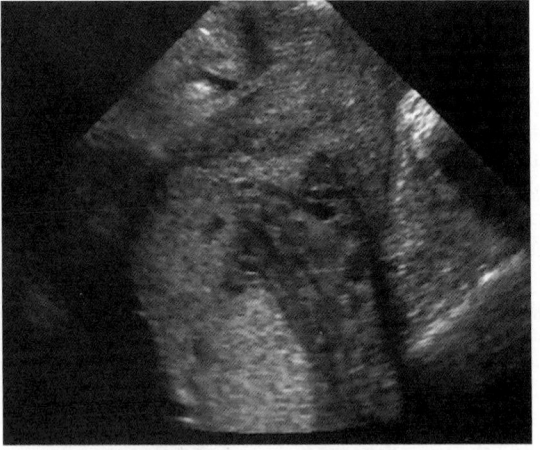

Labeled: **CERVIX TRANSLAB**

Amniotic Fluid

5. Depending on the stage of gestation, an overall longitudinal image of amniotic fluid or the largest pocket *with superior to inferior measurement.*

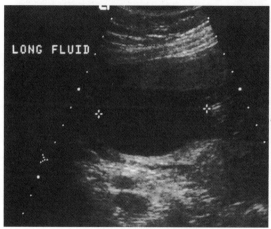

Labeled: **FLUID SAG**

SCANNING TIP: At times a quantitative measurement of amniotic fluid is required. Anteroposterior measurements are obtained for the right and left upper and lower quadrants. The sum of these anteroposterior measurements is called the amniotic fluid index. Fluid pockets that contain primarily cord or fetal parts are not included in the measurement.

6. Depending on the stage of gestation, an overall axial image of amniotic fluid or the largest pocket *with anterior to posterior and right to left measurements.*

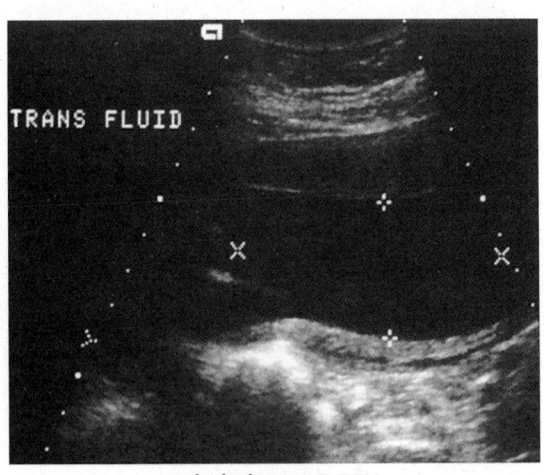

Labeled: **FLUID TRV**

SCANNING TIP: Because of the variability of fetal position and movement, the following fetal anatomy images may be taken in any sequence.

SCANNING TIP: An ultrasound examination during the second and third trimesters requires the documentation of a large number of anatomic structures; therefore two or more structures can be documented on a single image if they are well represented.

SCANNING TIP: Because of the variability of fetal position and movement, the scanning plane is not included as part of the film labeling for the following images.

Fetal Anatomy

7. Longitudinal image of the cervical spine.

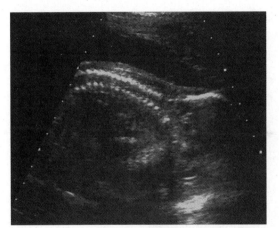

Labeled: **C SPINE**

8. Longitudinal image of the thoracic spine.

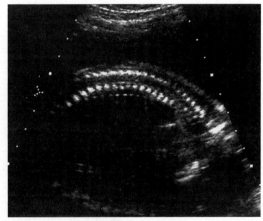

Labeled: **T SPINE**

PART V

9. Longitudinal image of the lumbar spine.

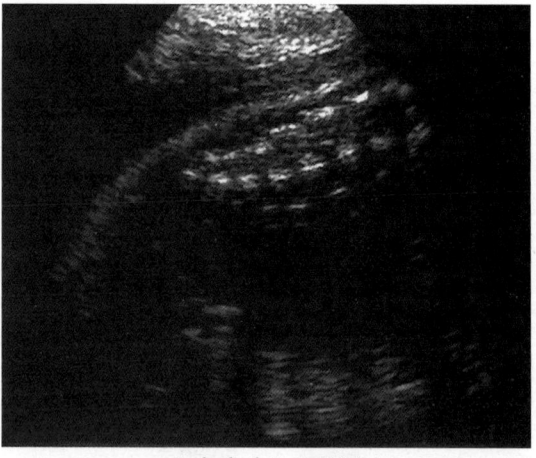

Labeled: **L SPINE**

10. Longitudinal image of the sacral spine.

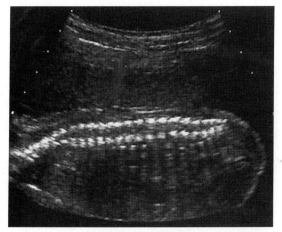

Labeled: **S SPINE**

SCANNING TIP: In some cases the long axis of the spine can be visualized on a single image. If so, take the image and label it as:
Labeled:
SPINE LONG AX

11. Axial image of the cervical spine.

Labeled: C SPINE

12. Axial image of the thoracic spine.

Labeled: T SPINE

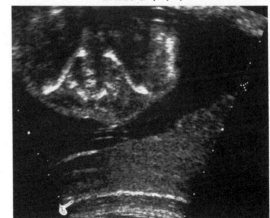

13. Axial image of the lumbar spine.

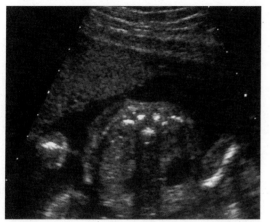

Labeled: **L SPINE**

14. 4-chamber view of the fetal heart to include its location within the thorax.

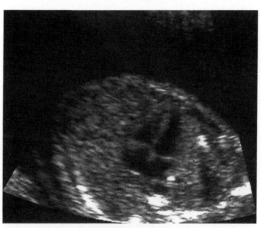

Labeled: **HEART**

15. Optional image showing the normal right ventricular outflow tract.

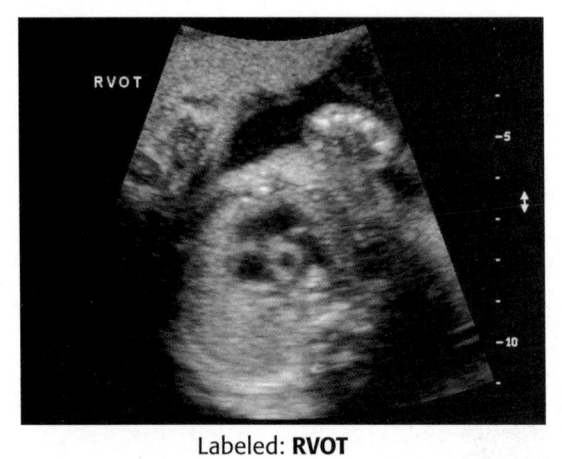

Labeled: **RVOT**

16. Optional image showing the normal left ventricular outflow tract.

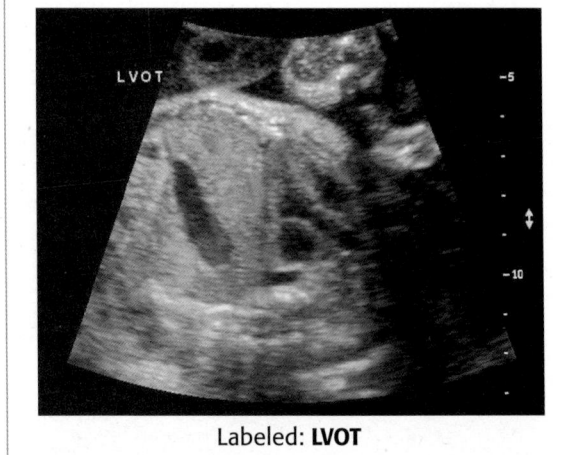

Labeled: **LVOT**

17. Axial image of fetal kidneys together.

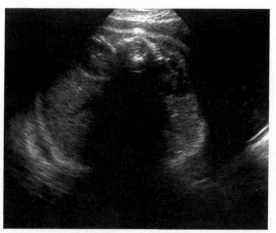

Labeled: **KIDNEYS**

SCANNING TIP: In cases where the kidneys cannot be imaged together because of fetal position or movement, take separate axial images of each kidney and label accordingly.

18. Longitudinal image of the right kidney.

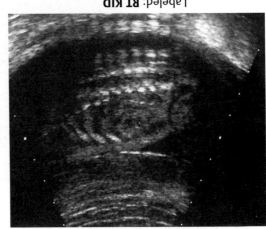

Labeled: **RT KID**

19. Longitudinal image of the left kidney.

Labeled: **LT KID**

20. Image of the urinary bladder.

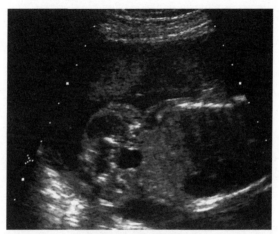

Labeled: **UR BLADDER**

21. Image of the umbilical cord insertion site on the anterior abdominal wall.

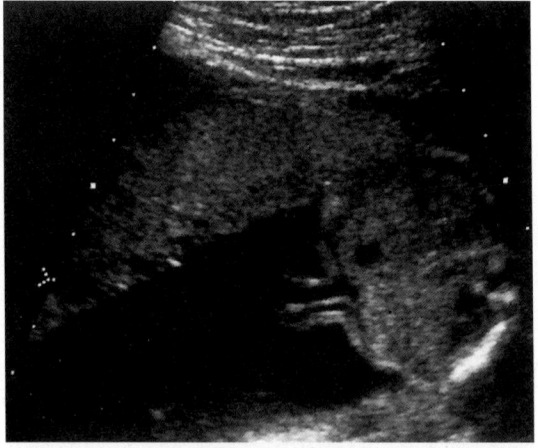

Labeled: **CORD**

SCANNING TIP: If the insertion site image does not distinguish the three vessels of the cord, take an additional image of the cord to demonstrate the three vessels and label accordingly.

22. A magnified view of an axial section of the 3-vessel umbilical cord.

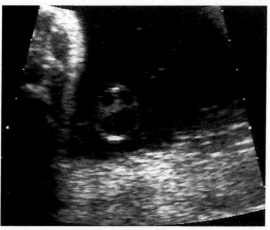

Labeled: **CORD**

23. Image of the stomach if visualized.

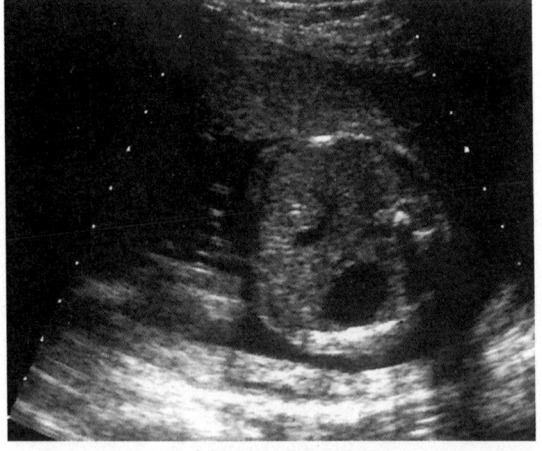

Labeled: **STOMACH**

SCANNING TIP: The image of the stomach is not necessary if the stomach was documented on any other image.

24. Image of genitalia.

a. Image of male genitalia.

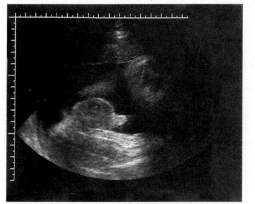

Labeled: **GENITALIA**

b. Image of female genitalia.

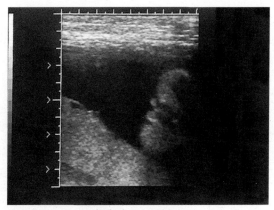

Labeled: **GENITALIA**

25. Longitudinal image of the fetus to include the diaphragm.

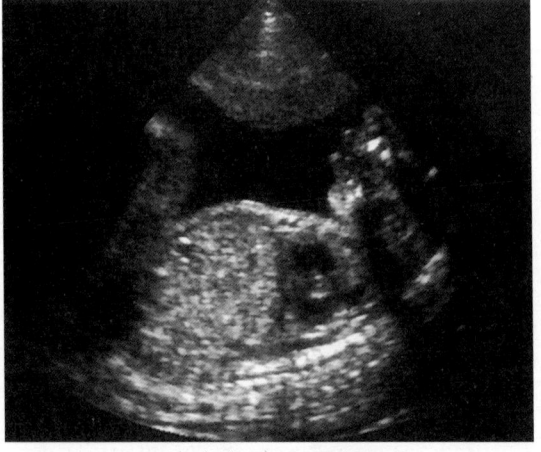

Labeled: **DIAPHRAGM**

26. Biparietal diameter image at the level of the thalamus and the cavum septum pellucidi. *Measurement is from the outside of the near cranium to the inside of the far cranium (leading edge to leading edge).*

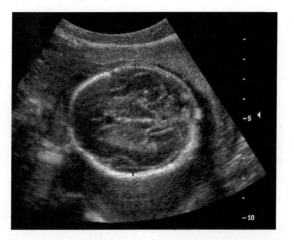

SCANNING TIP: Because of the obvious nature of the fetal measurements, specifics are not included as part of the film labeling for the following measurement images.

27. Cerebellum with measurement.

28. Cisterna magnum with measurement.

29. Nuchal fold (done between 16 and 24 weeks) *with measurement.*

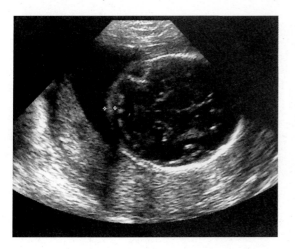

SCANNING TIP: The measurement of the nuchal fold is not always routinely performed but should be considered for the fetus of mothers over 35 years of age or when the mother has a lower-than-normal serum alpha-fetoprotein level. The extra fold of soft tissue visualized at the back of the neck is considered a sonographic marker for the second trimester detection of Down syndrome.

30. Head circumference image at the same level as the biparietal diameter or use the biparietal diameter image. *Measurement is around the outline of the cranium.* Up-to-date ultrasound equipment provides tracking balls to trace the cranium or calipers that open to outline the cranium.

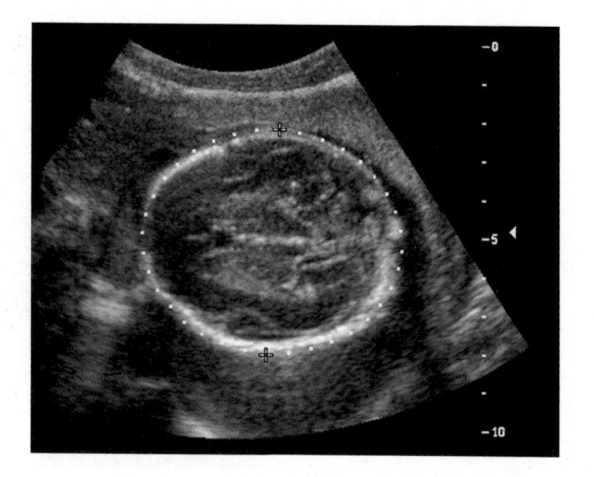

31. Image of the choroid plexus.

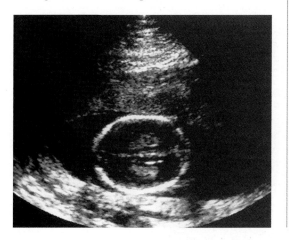

32. Lateral ventricle *with measurement*.

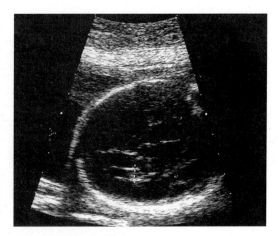

33. Abdominal circumference image at the level of the junction of the umbilical vein and portal vein sinus. *Measurement is around the outline of the abdomen.* The abdomen should appear round.

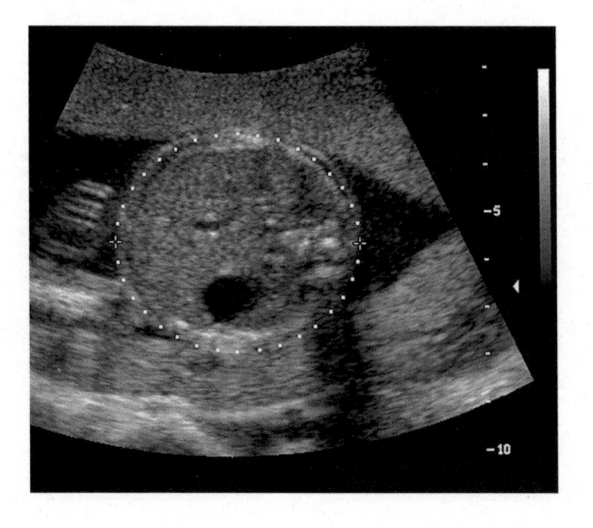

34. Long axis image of the femur *with measurement from one ossified end of the femur to the other ossified end.*

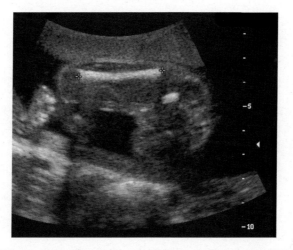

SCANNING TIP: For long bone measurements, cursors are placed at the bone-cartilage interface. The cartilaginous ends of the bones are not included in the measurement.

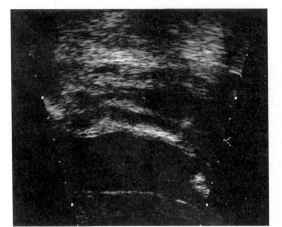

36. Image of the lower portion of the leg.

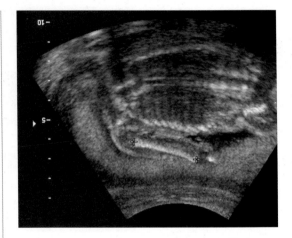

35. Long axis image of the humerus with measurement from one ossified end of the humerus to the other ossified end.

37. Image of the radius and ulna.

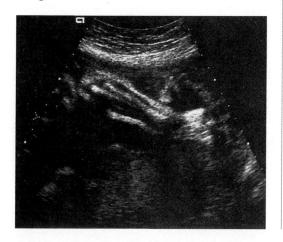

38. Image of a hand.

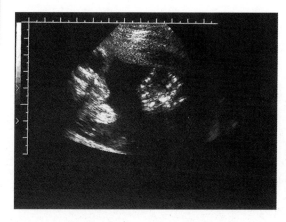

39. Another image of the hand.

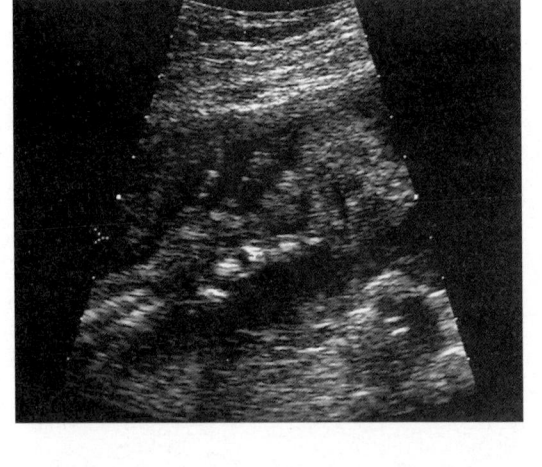

40. Image of facial profile.

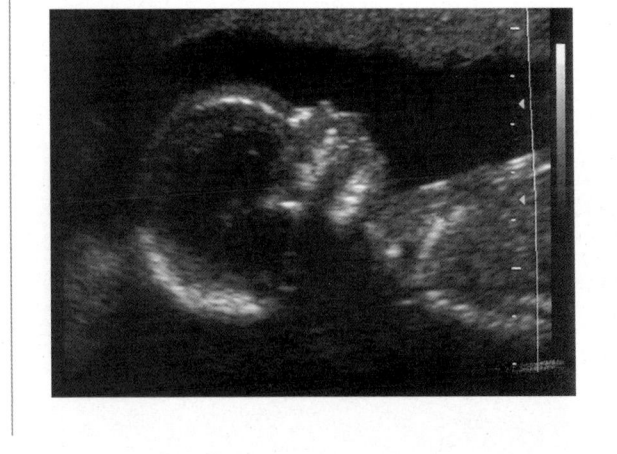

41. Coronal image of the nostrils and lips.

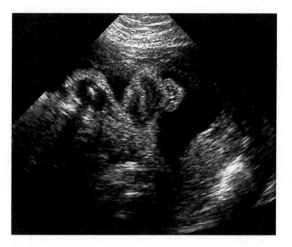

SCANNING TIP: Most physicians only require images of one hand, foot, arm, and leg based on the assumption that both were evaluated during the survey.

SECTION FOUR ▪ Image Protocol for the Sonographic Study of Multiple Gestations

Criteria

- In addition to the required images for multiple gestations, each fetus of a multiple gestation should be imaged as previously described for singleton pregnancies.
- No limited studies.
- Before the examination, a patient history including the date of the first day of the patient's last period, gravidity, parity, and history of any pelvic surgery should be taken.
- Begin multiple gestation studies with a survey of the uterus and adnexa followed by the pregnancies.
- When transvaginal or translabial sonography is used in conjunction with the routine transabdominal study, the patient's verbal or written consent is required. Also, the examination should be chaperoned by a female health care professional, whose initials should be included as part of the film labeling.
- Do not share study results with the patient. Legally, only physicians can give a diagnosis.

Multiple Gestations Study

Gestational Sacs

Each fetus of a multiple gestation should be imaged as previously described for single-ton pregnancies plus the following additional views as they apply:
1. Image of a twin pregnancy demonstrating separate sacs.

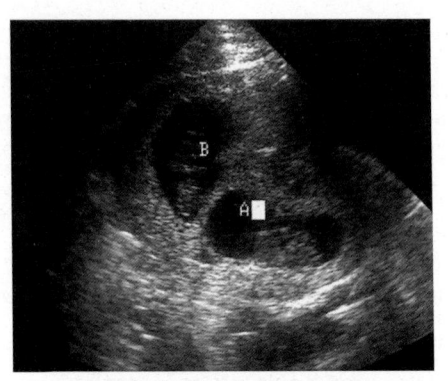

Labeled: **TWINS/SEP SACS**

2. Image of second trimester twins demonstrating the presence of a separating membrane.

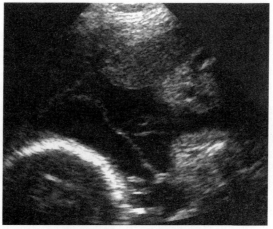

Labeled: **TWINS/MEMBRANE**

3. Image of triplets.

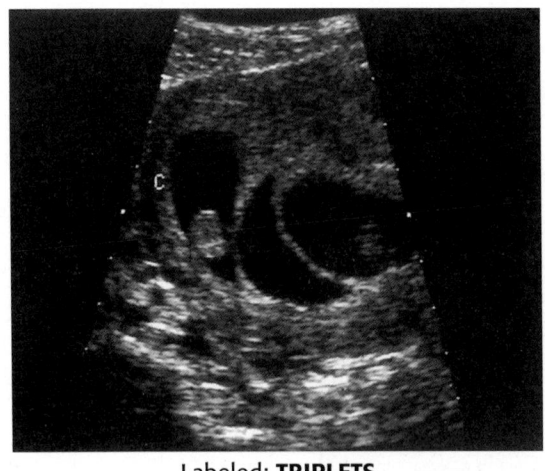

Labeled: **TRIPLETS**

SCANNING TIP: It is important to demonstrate the position of the presenting fetus. This is the fetus that is lower in the uterus, closer to the cervix, and will be delivered first. This fetus is labeled "a" and the other fetus is labeled "b." If there are more than two (as in number 3), then "c," "d," etc. will be used. This labeling allows individual growth rates to be determined. If possible, determine the gender of each fetus. This information may help determine whether they are fraternal or identical.

The Biophysical Profile

During the late third trimester the biophysical profile is often obtained. This test measures fetal well-being and consists of five parameters. The first part of the test involves a nonstress test. This test is performed in the delivery room or in an obstetrician's office and measures spontaneous heart rate accelerations. This part of the biophysical profile is not performed by the sonographer. The remaining four parameters, measured by the sonographer, are (1) fluid, (2) fetal respiration, (3) fetal tone, and (4) gross body motion. These parameters and the scoring system are described in Table 5-1.

Table 5-1 Biophysical Profile Scoring

	Criterion	Score (Pts)
Part I		
Nonstress Test	2 accelerations of 15 beats/min in 30-min examination	2
Part II: Ultrasound Examination		
Gross movement	3 separate flexions and extensions in 30-min examination	2
Tone	1 episode of fetal opening and closing of hand or clenching of foot in 30-min examination	2
Respiration	At least 60 sec of fetal breathing in 30-min examination	2
Fluid	At least one pocket of amniotic fluid of at least 1 cm in 2 dimensions	2
	Unqualified pass	8 or more
	Maximum total	10

Data from Manning EA, Platt LD, Sipos L: Antenatal fetal evaluation: development of a fetal biophysical profile. *Am J Obstet Gynecol.* 1980;136:787-795.

Amniotic Fluid

1. Demonstration of a pocket of fluid.

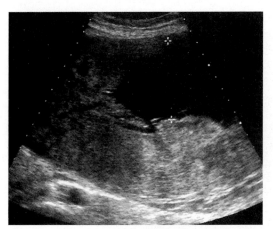

Labeled: **FLUID**

2. Demonstration of fetal respiration.

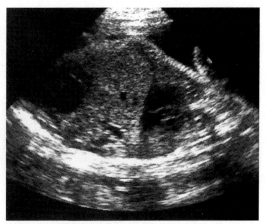

Labeled: **DIAPHRAGM/RESP**

3. Demonstration of fetal tone.

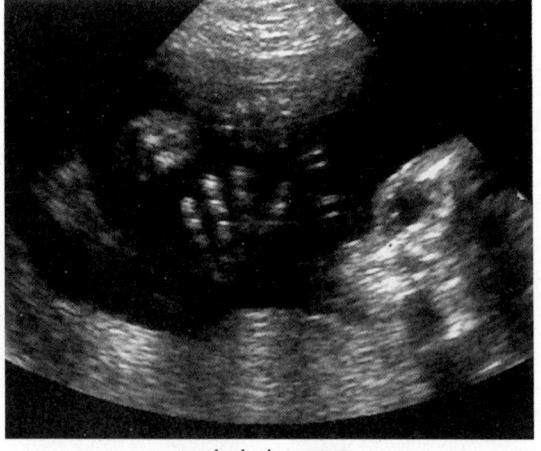

Labeled: **HAND**

4. Demonstration of FETAL GROSS BODY MOTION.

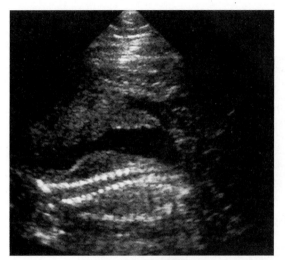

Labeled: **MOTION**

SCANNING TIP: Occasionally it is necessary to measure the resistance to blood flow within the umbilical arteries. This measurement is obtained by interrogating the umbilical cord artery with low power Doppler. The ratio of the peak systolic flow to the end diastolic flow is calculated (SD ratio). This number varies with the age of the fetus and charts are available to determine if blood flow through the cord is adequate.

5. Umbilical artery Doppler measurement and determination of the SD ratio.

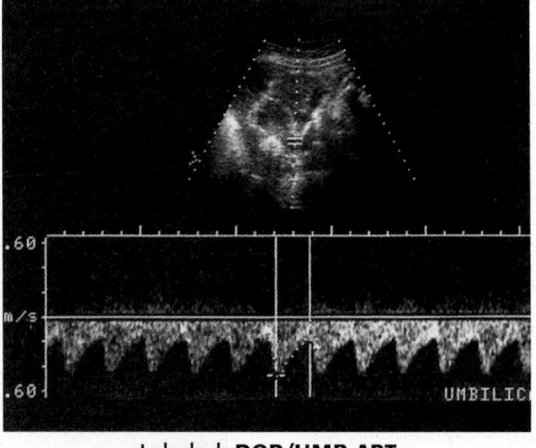

Labeled: **DOP/UMB ART**

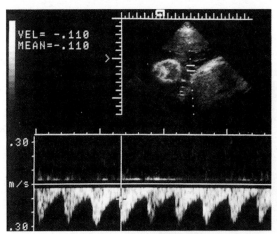

VEL= -.110
MEAN=-.110

.30

m/s

.30

Labeled: **DOP/UMB ART**

SCANNING TIP: In some cases, the physician may also want to determine if blood flow to the placenta from the mother's circulation is adequate, so another Doppler measurement is made at the interface between the placenta and uterus or in the uterine artery if possible. The SD ratio for the Doppler waveform is calculated and checked against a chart value for the appropriate gestational age.

6. Uterine artery Doppler measurement and determination of the SD ratio.

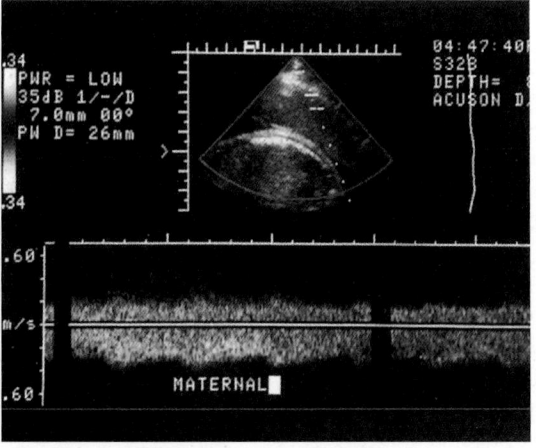

Labeled: **DOP/UT AR**

SMALL PARTS

SECTION ONE ▪ Image Protocol for the Sonographic Study of the Musculoskeletal System

Criteria

- Begin studies with a survey of structures in at least 2 scanning planes.
- Do not share study results with the patient. Legally, only physicians can give a diagnosis.

Musculoskeletal Study (Rotator Cuff, Carpal Tunnel, and Achilles Tendon)

Rotator Cuff Study

1. Axial image of the bicep tendon.

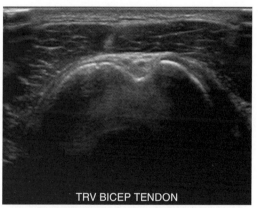

TRV BICEP TENDON

Labeled: **(RT or LT) BT TRV**

2. Longitudinal image of the bicep tendon.

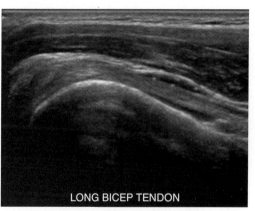

LONG BICEP TENDON

Labeled: **(RT or LT) BT SAG**

PART VI

3. Long axis image of the subscapularis tendon.

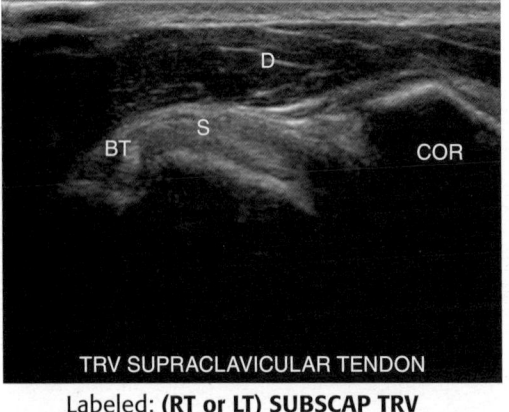

TRV SUPRACLAVICULAR TENDON

Labeled: **(RT or LT) SUBSCAP TRV**

4. Axial image of the subscapularis tendon.

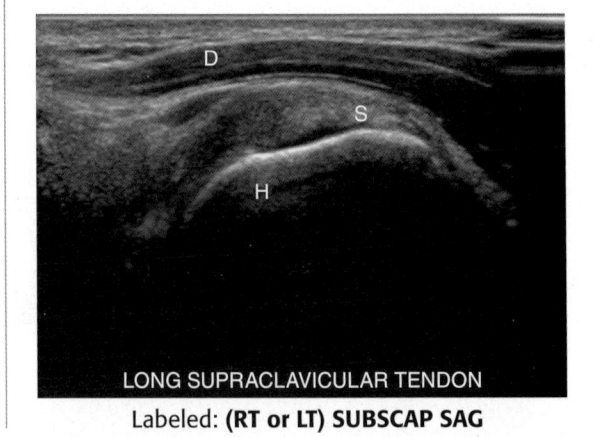

LONG SUPRACLAVICULAR TENDON

Labeled: **(RT or LT) SUBSCAP SAG**

5. Long axis image of the supraspinatus tendon.

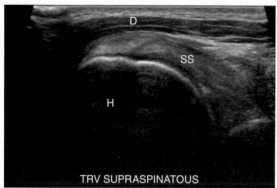

TRV SUPRASPINATOUS

Labeled: **(RT or LT) SUPRASPIN TRV**

6. Axial image of the supraspinatus tendon.

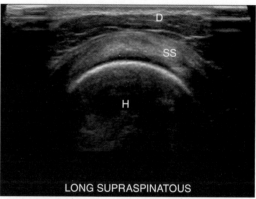

LONG SUPRASPINATOUS

Labeled: **(RT or LT) SUPRASPIN SAG**

7. Axial image of the infraspinatous tendon.

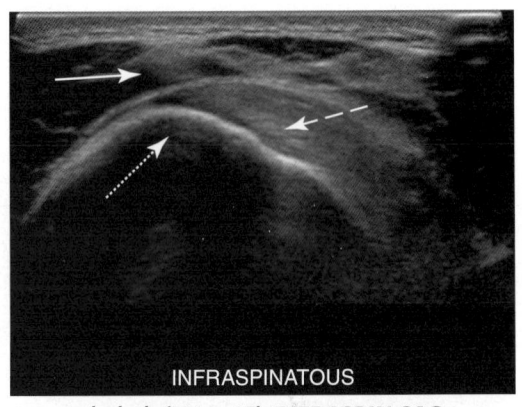

INFRASPINATOUS

Labeled: **(RT or LT) INFRASPIN SAG**

8. Long axis image of the infraspinatous tendon.

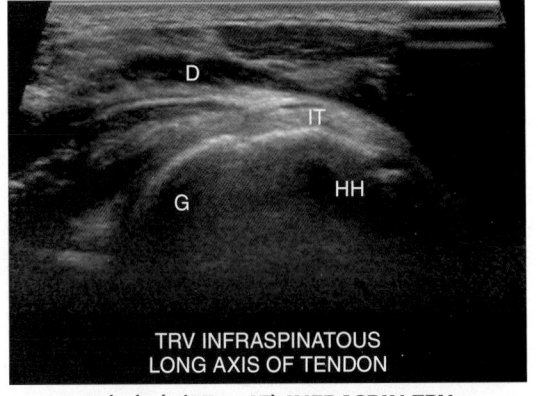

TRV INFRASPINATOUS
LONG AXIS OF TENDON

Labeled: **(RT or LT) INFRASPIN TRV**

9. Long axis image of the teres minor tendon.

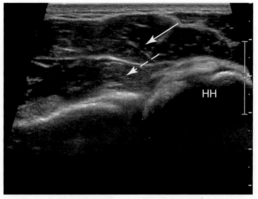

Labeled: **(RT OR LT) TM TRV**

10. Axial image of the teres minor tendon.

Labeled: **(RT OR LT) TM SAG**

Carpal Tunnel Study

1. Transverse image of the proximal carpal tunnel. (*Dashed arrow*, median nerve; *dash-dotted arrow*, flexor superficialis tendon; *solid arrow*, flexor profundus tendon)

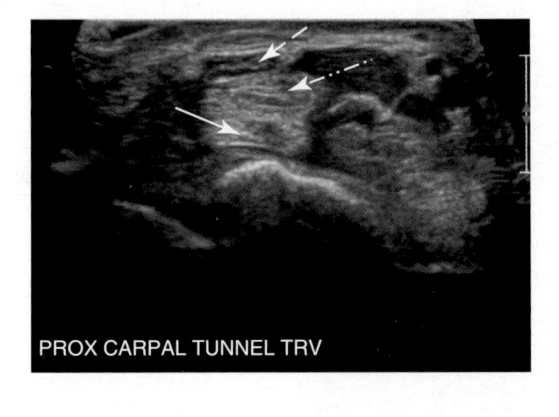

2. Transverse image of the distal carpal tunnel. (*MN*, median nerve)

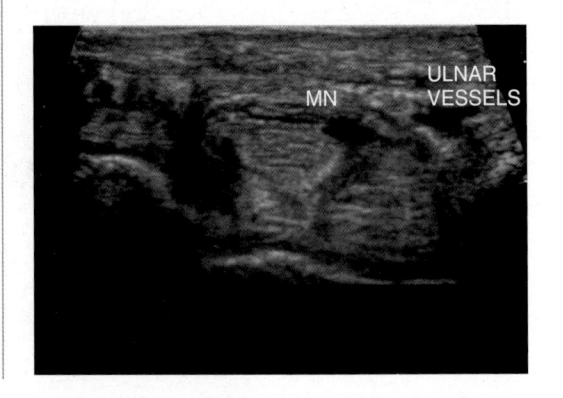

3. Sagittal image of the proximal carpal tunnel. (*Dashed arrow*, median nerve; *dash-dotted arrow*, flexor superficialis tendon; *solid arrow*, flexor profundus tendon)

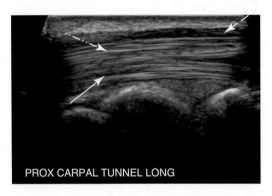

PROX CARPAL TUNNEL LONG

4. Sagittal image of the distal carpal tunnel. (*Dashed arrow*, median nerve; *solid arrow*, flexor superficialis tendon; *dotted arrow*, flexor profundus tendon)

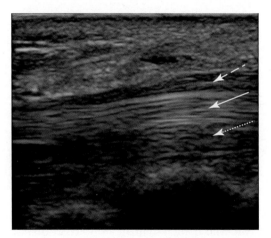

Achilles Tendon Study

1. Long axis of the Achilles tendon at the insertion point. (Arrow: Achilles tendon)

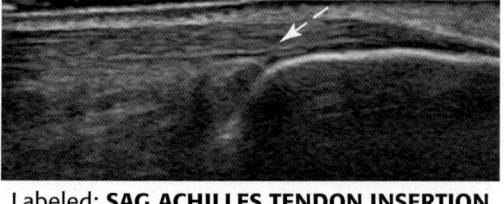

Labeled: **SAG ACHILLES TENDON INSERTION POINT**

2. Long axis of the Achilles tendon proximally just superior to the point of insertion.

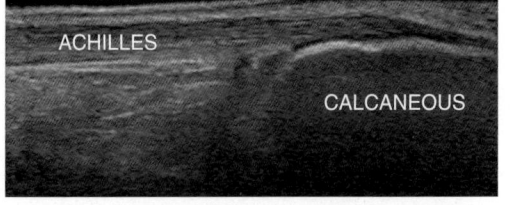

Labeled: **SAG ACHILLES TENDON PROX**

3. Long axis of the mid-Achilles tendon.

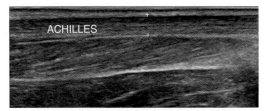

Labeled: **SAG ACHILLES TENDON MID**

4. Long axis of the distal Achilles tendon.
   (*Arrow*: Achilles tendon)

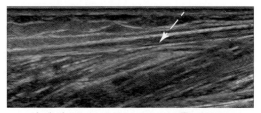

Labeled: **SAG ACHILLES TENDON DISTAL**

5. Panoramic view of entire length of Achilles tendon.

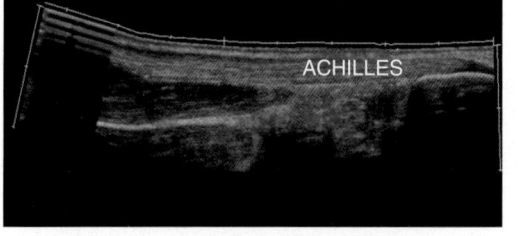

Labeled: **SAG ACHILLES TENDON**

6. Transverse axis of Achilles tendon at insertion point.

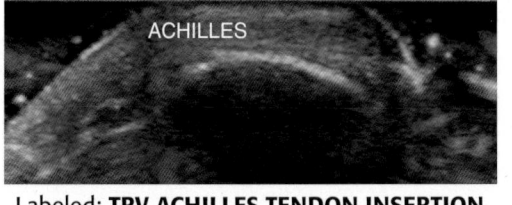

Labeled: **TRV ACHILLES TENDON INSERTION**

7. Transverse axis of Achilles tendon proximally just superior to insertion point.

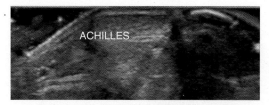

Labeled: **TRV ACHILLES TENDON PROX**

8. Transverse axis of mid-Achilles tendon.

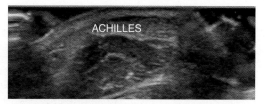

Labeled: **TRV ACHILLES TENDON MID**

9. Transverse axis of Achilles tendon distal.

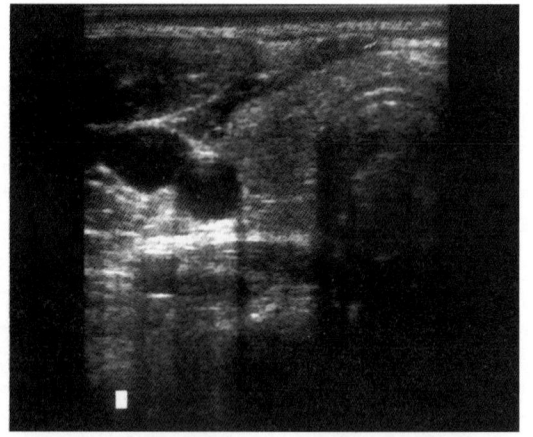

Labeled: **TRV ACHILLES TENDON DISTAL**

SECTION TWO ▪ Image Protocol for the Sonographic Study of the Thyroid Gland

PART VI

Criteria

Begin studies with a survey of the thyroid gland and associated structures in at least 2 scanning planes.

- As a general rule, the parathyroid glands are not appreciated sonographically unless they are abnormal.
- Do not share study results with the patient. Legally, only physicians can give a diagnosis.

Thyroid Gland Study

Thyroid • Right Lobe • Axial Images

1. Axial image of the inferior portion of the right lobe.

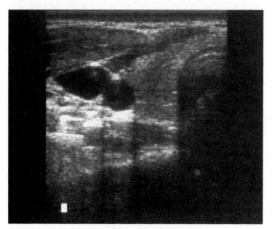

Labeled: **RT LOBE TRV INF**

2. Axial image of the midportion of the right lobe.

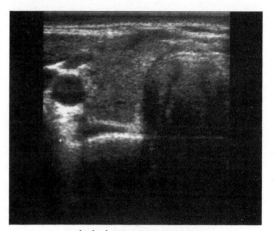

Labeled: **RT LOBE TRV MID**

PART VI

Labeled: RT LOBE TRV SUP

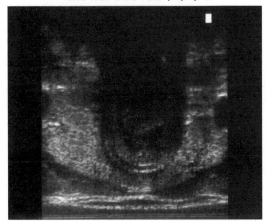

3. Axial image of the superior portion of the right lobe.

Labeled: ISTHMUS TRV

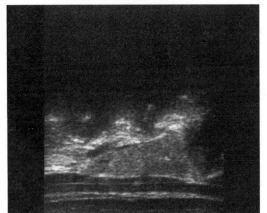

4. Longitudinal image of the isthmus to include both the right and left lobe attachments.

Thyroid • Right Lobe • Longitudinal Images

5. Longitudinal image of the medial portion of the right lobe.

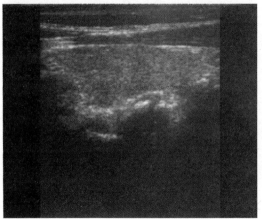

Labeled: **RT LOBE SAG MED**

6. Longitudinal image of the lateral portion of the right lobe.

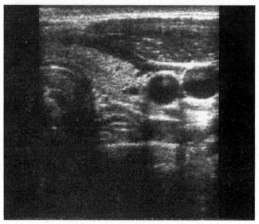

Labeled: **RT LOBE SAG LAT**

Thyroid • Left Lobe • Axial Images

7. Axial image of the inferior portion of the left lobe.

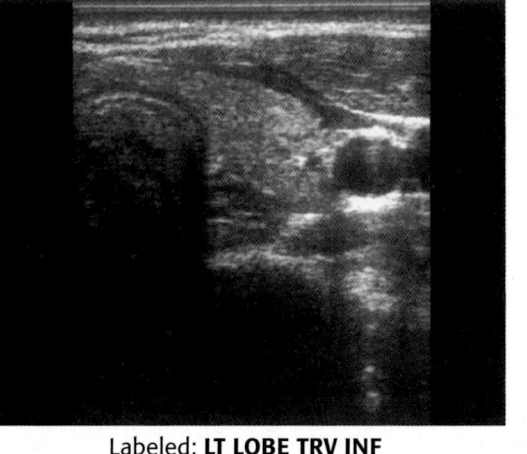

Labeled: **LT LOBE TRV INF**

8. Axial image of the midportion of the left lobe.

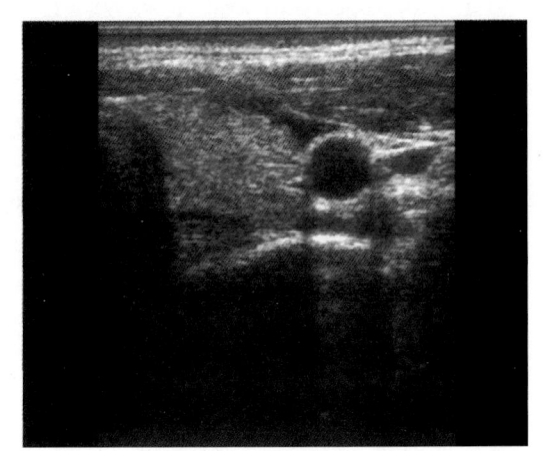

Labeled: **LT LOBE TRV MID**

9. Axial image of the superior portion of the left lobe.

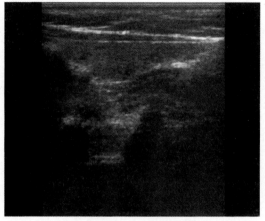

Labeled: **LT LOBE TRV SUP**

Thyroid • Left Lobe • Longitudinal Images

10. Longitudinal image of the medial portion of the left lobe.

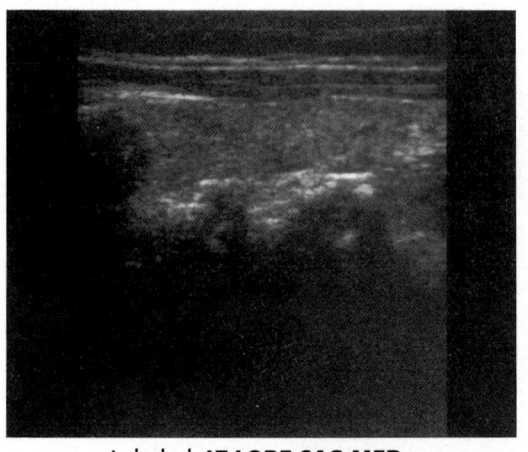

Labeled: **LT LOBE SAG MED**

11. Longitudinal image of the lateral portion of the left lobe.

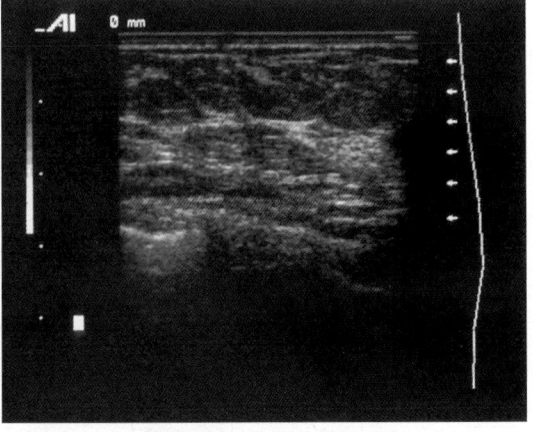

Labeled: **LT LOBE SAG LAT**

SECTION THREE ▪ Image Protocols for the Sonographic Study of the Breast

Criteria

- In most cases, for women under 30 and lactating and pregnant women, breast sonography has become the first phase of imaging for evaluating palpable masses. Breast sonography, however, is not recognized as a screening study for microcalcifications.
- Breast sonography is generally performed to determine the composition or characterization of a localized lesion or lesions (that may or may not be palpable) and to further evaluate mammographic and clinical findings.
- Additional indications for breast sonography include guidance for biopsies, treatment plan for radiation therapy, and evaluating complications associated with breast implants.
- In some cases, whole breast scanning may be recommended for diffuse diseases such as fibrocystic disease.
- Begin studies with a survey of the structure(s) in at least two scanning planes.

- Do not share study results with the patient. Legally, only physicians can give diagnoses.
- Use the following image of normal breast tissue as a technical guideline. Remember that the thickness of the sonographically distinct layers of the breast varies with age.

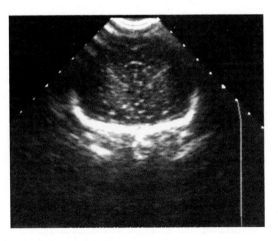

Breast Lesion Characterization

SCANNING TIP: The location of the lesion must be recorded to accompany the required images.

The location of the lesion can be indicated by one of the following methods:
- Showing it on a diagram of the breast
- Specifying the quadrant
- Using clock notation and distance from the nipple.

SCANNING TIP: Image labeling should include right or left breast, lesion location, and transducer orientation with regard to the breast (axial or longitudinal, radial or antiradial).

Breast Lesion • Right Breast or Left Breast • Longitudinal Images

1. Longitudinal image of the lesion with measurement from the most superior to the most inferior margin.

   Labeled: **SITE LOCATION AND SCANNING PLANE**

2. Same image as number 1 without measurement calipers.

   Labeled: **SITE LOCATION AND SCANNING PLANE**

Breast Lesion • Right Breast or Left Breast • Axial Images

3. Axial image of the lesion with measurements from the most anterior to the most posterior margin and from the most lateral to lateral or lateral to medial margin.

   Labeled: **SITE LOCATION AND SCANNING PLANE**

4. Same image as number 3 without measurement calipers.

   Labeled: **SITE LOCATION AND SCANNING PLANE**

Breast Lesion • Right Breast or Left Breast • Longitudinal and Axial High and Low Gain Images

5. Longitudinal image of the lesion with high gain technique.

   Labeled: **SITE LOCATION, SCANNING PLANE, HIGH GAIN**

6. Axial image of the lesion with high gain technique.

   Labeled: **SITE LOCATION, SCANNING PLANE, HIGH GAIN**

7. Longitudinal image of the lesion with low gain technique.

   Labeled: **SITE LOCATION, SCANNING PLANE, LOW GAIN**

8. Axial image of the lesion with low gain technique.

   Labeled: **SITE LOCATION, SCANNING PLANE, LOW GAIN**

SCANNING TIP: Depending on the size and complexity of the lesion, additional images (in at least two scanning planes) may be necessary to document the extent of the lesion.

Whole Breast Study

Whole Breast Images • Right Breast or Left Breast

1. 12 o'clock image of breast tissue with the base of the transducer toward the nipple and the end of the transducer facing outward so that the nipple area is closest to the top of the imaging screen.

   Labeled: **12 O'CLOCK RT LT**

2. 3 o'clock image (same orientation as number 1).

   Labeled: **3 O'CLOCK RT LT**

3. 6 o'clock image.

   Labeled: **6 O'CLOCK RT LT**

4. 9 o'clock image.

   Labeled: **9 O'CLOCK RT LT**

5. Axial image through the nipple.

   Labeled: **NIP TRV RT LT**

6. Longitudinal image through the nipple.

   Labeled: **NIP SAG RT LT**

7. Longitudinal image of the axillary region.

   Labeled: **AXILLARY SAG RT LT**

8. Axial image of the axillary region.

   Labeled: **AXILLARY TRV RT LT**

9 to 16. The same corresponding images of the other breast.

SCANNING TIP: In some cases, whole breast scanning includes images from 12 o'clock, 1 o'clock, 2 o'clock, 3 o'clock, etc. If so, label accordingly and include nipple and axillary images.

SECTION FOUR ▪ Image Protocol for the Sonographic Study of the Neonatal Brain

Criteria

- Begin studies with a survey of the brain in at least 2 scanning planes.
- Infants should be kept warm and disturbed as little as possible.
- Do not share study results with the patient. Legally, only physicians can give diagnoses.

Coronal Images

1. Coronal image of the frontal lobes of the brain with the interhemispheric fissure. Include the orbital cones and ethmoid sinus.

2. Coronal image of the frontal horns of the ventricles encompassing the caudate nucleus. Include the germinal matrix adjacent to the ventricles and corpus callosum.

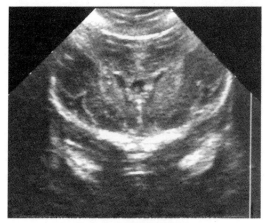

Labeled: **CORONAL**

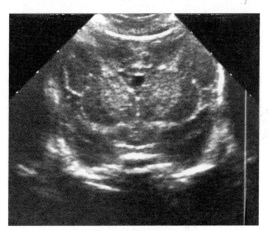

Labeled: **CORONAL**

3. Coronal image of the frontal horns and thalami. Include the Sylvian fissures, septum pellucidum, third ventricle, and foramen of Monro.

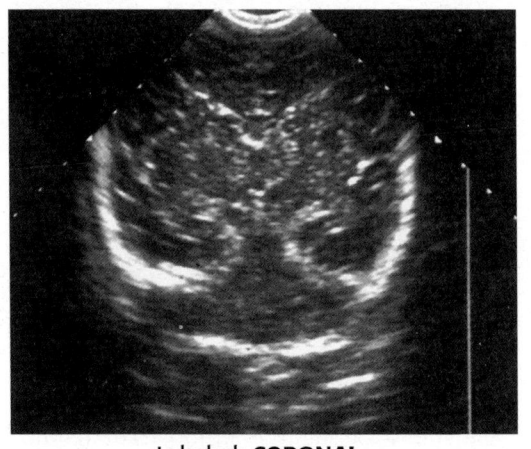

Labeled: **CORONAL**

4. Coronal image of the bodies of the lateral ventricles, thalami, Sylvian fissures, choroidal fissures, and temporal horns.

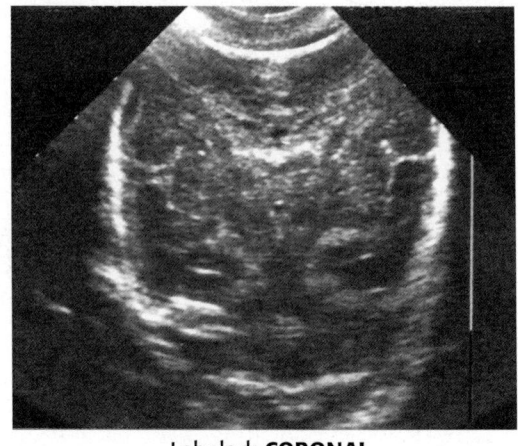

Labeled: **CORONAL**

5. Coronal image of the tentorium cerebelli. Include the Sylvian fissures and the cisterna magna.

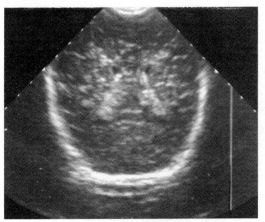

Labeled: **CORONAL**

6. Coronal image of the choroid plexus in the atrium or trigone region.

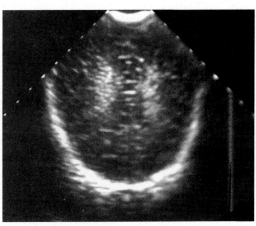

Labeled: **CORONAL**

7. Coronal image of the occipital lobes of the brain.

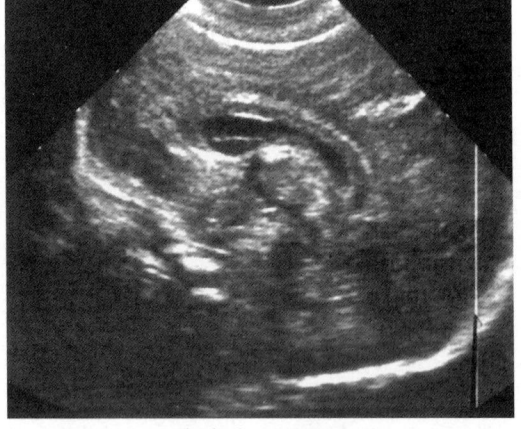

Labeled: **CORONAL**

Sagittal Images

8. Sagittal midline image of the cavum septum pellucidum, corpus callosum, third ventricle, fourth ventricle, and cerebellum, including the massa intermedia (seen in two thirds of infants).

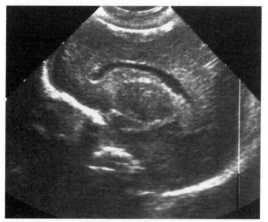

Labeled: **SAG ML**

SCANNING TIP: This image should be perpendicular at the midline.

9. Sagittal image of the right ventricle, germinal matrix, caudate nucleus, thalamus, and choroid plexus.

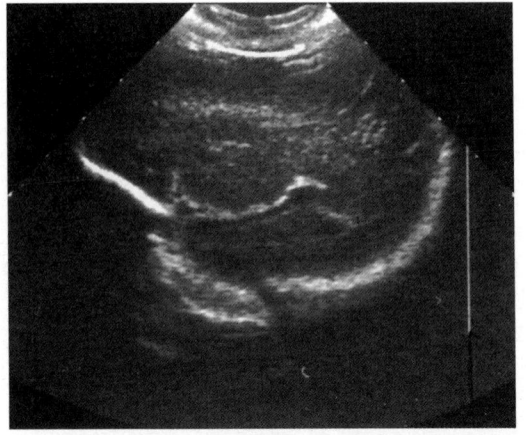

Labeled: **SAG RT LAT**

SCANNING TIP: In some cases the frontal horn, body, temporal horn, and occipital horn cannot be imaged in the same plane. Therefore an additional image(s) may be necessary.

10. Sagittal image of the right temporal lobe of the brain at the level of the Sylvian fissure.

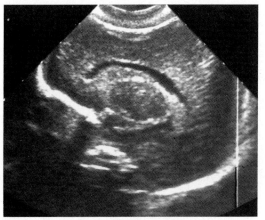

Labeled: **SAG RT LAT**

11. Sagittal image of the left ventricle, germinal matrix, caudate nucleus, thalamus, and choroid plexus.

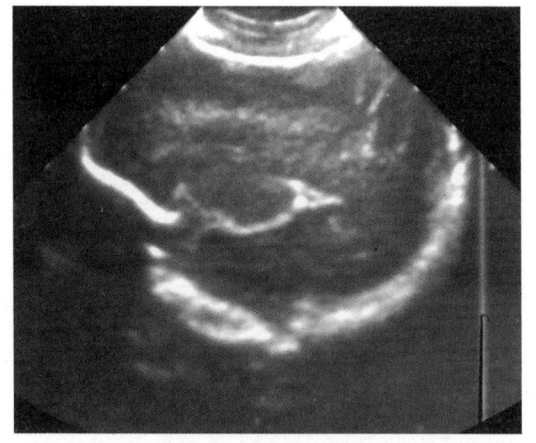

Labeled: **SAG LT LAT**

SCANNING TIP: In some cases the frontal horn, body, temporal horn, and occipital horn cannot be imaged in the same plane. Therefore an additional image(s) may be necessary.

12. Sagittal image of the left temporal lobe of the brain at the level of the Sylvian fissure.

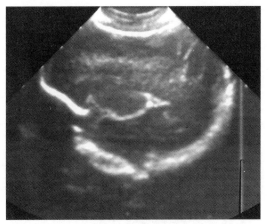

Labeled: **SAG LT LAT**

SCANNING TIP: Alternative axial views through the temporal recess or posterior fontanelle are options to further evaluate the lateral ventricular walls and/or the occipital horns, respectively.

VASCULAR SYSTEM

SECTION ONE ▪ Image Protocols for Abdominal Doppler and Color Flow Studies

Criteria

- Do not share the results of the study with the patient. Legally, only physicians can give a diagnosis.

Mesenteric Arterial Study*

1. Longitudinal image of the aorta at level of celiac artery origin.

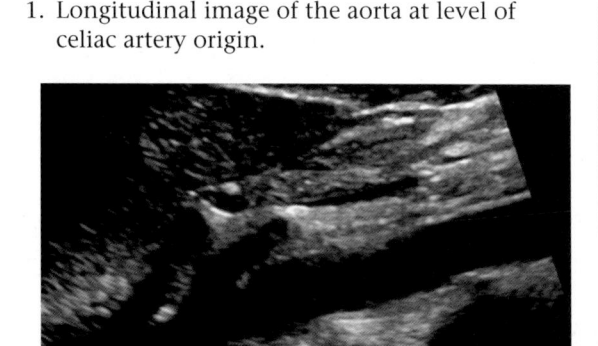

Labeled: **SAG AORTA CELIAC ORIGIN**

2. Doppler spectral waveform from the celiac artery origin.

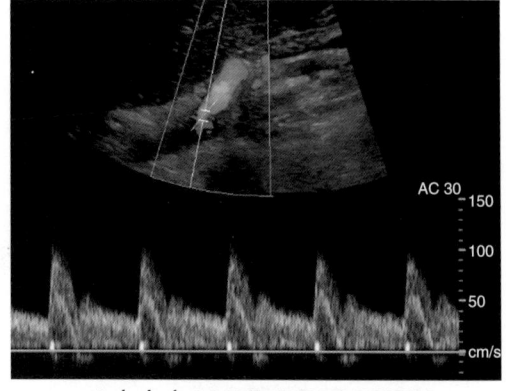

Labeled: **AORTA CELIAC ORIGIN**

---

*Mesenteric images courtesy Penn State Hershey Vascular Noninvasive Diagnostic Laboratory, Hershey, Pa.

3. Doppler spectral waveform from the distal celiac trunk.

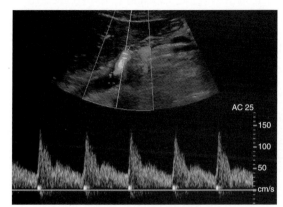

Labeled: **CELIAC DIST**

4. Axial image of the aorta demonstrating longitudinal sections of the celiac artery and the common hepatic and splenic arteries at the celiac bifurcation.

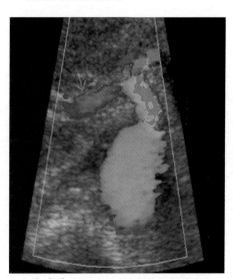

Labeled: **TRV CELIAC BIFURCATION**

5. Doppler spectral waveforms from the common hepatic (**A**) and splenic arteries **(B).**

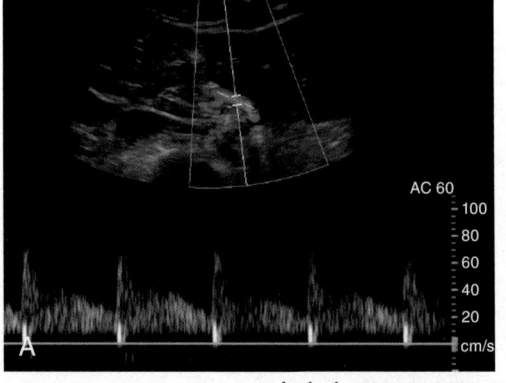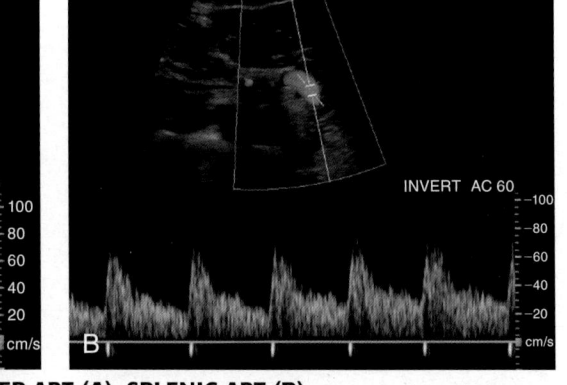

Labeled: **COMM HEP ART (A), SPLENIC ART (B)**

SCANNING TIP: The hepatic artery may be followed from the celiac artery bifurcation to the level of its entry into the liver at the porta hepatis. Images and Doppler spectral waveforms should be documented throughout the proximal, mid, and distal segments of the vessel. In a similar manner, the splenic artery may be examined from its origin at the celiac bifurcation to the level of the splenic hilum. Images and Doppler spectral waveforms are documented throughout the proximal, mid, and distal segments of the vessel. The splenic artery is frequently quite tortuous and color flow imaging may facilitate examination of this artery.

6. Longitudinal image of the SMA from its origin to its midsection.

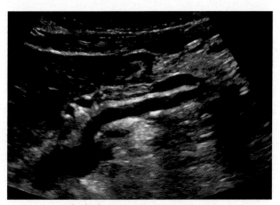

Labeled: **SAG SMA PROX-MID**

7. Doppler spectral waveforms from the proximal to mid **SMA.**

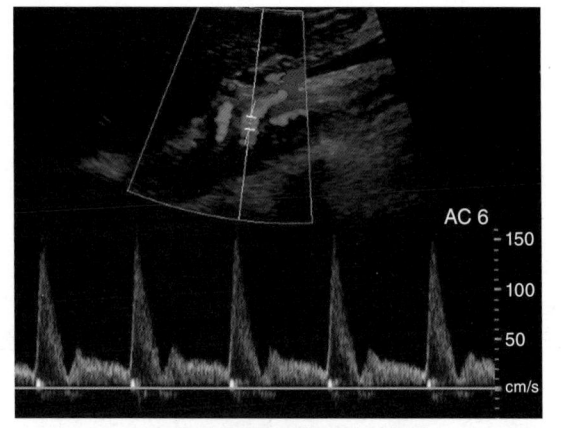

Labeled: **SMA PROX or MID**

SCANNING TIP: The inferior mesenteric artery (IMA) is not routinely examined. If the celiac and/or SMA are critically stenosed or occluded, the IMA would be evaluated in a manner similar to the study of the SMA. At present, there are no well-validated diagnostic criteria for the IMA, but the presence of poststenotic turbulence would be suggestive of a hemodynamically significant lesion.

Renal Arterial Study*

1. Longitudinal image of the mid aorta.

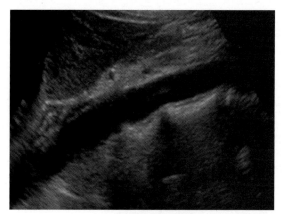

Labeled: **SAG AO**

2. Axial image of the aorta at the level of the left renal vein and origin of the renal arteries.

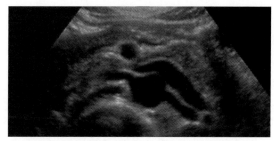

Labeled: **TRV ORIGIN RT and/or LT REN ART**

*Renal arterial images courtesy Penn State Hershey Vascular Noninvasive Diagnostic Laboratory, Hershey, Pa.

PART VII

3. Transition waveforms from the origin of the right or left renal artery.

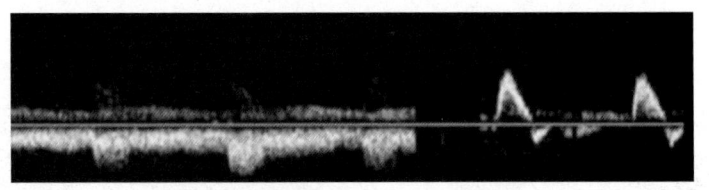

Labeled: **ORIGIN RT or LT REN ART**

4. Longitudinal image of proximal-to-mid right or left renal artery.

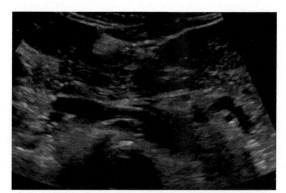

Labeled: **TRV RT or LT REN ART PROX-MID**

5. Doppler spectral waveforms from the proximal and mid segments of the renal artery.

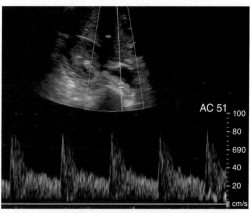

Labeled: **RT or LT REN ART PROX-MID**

6. Axial view of the kidney demonstrating the longitudinal section of the distal-to-mid segments of the renal artery.

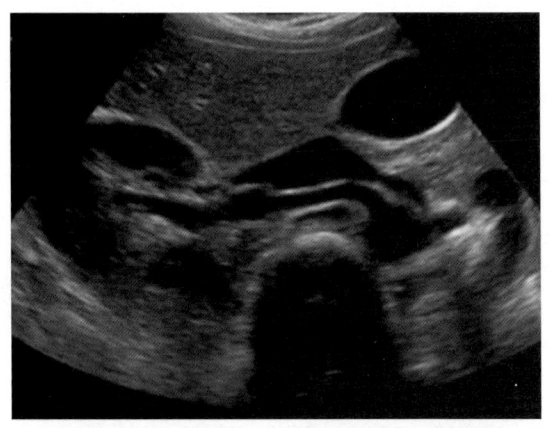

Labeled: **TRV RT or LT REN ART DIST-MID**

7. Doppler spectral waveforms from the distal and mid segments of the renal artery.

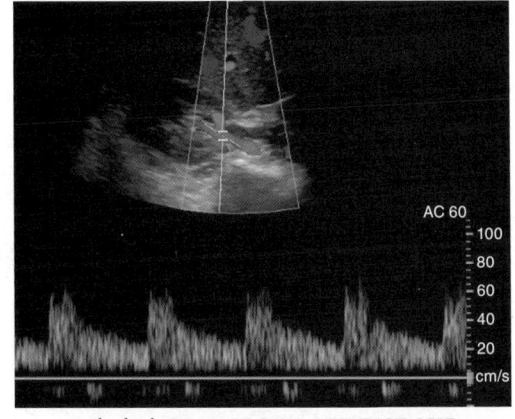

Labeled: **RT or LT REN ART DIST-MID**

8. Long axis image of the kidney *with measurement.*

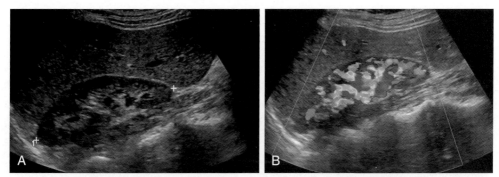

Labeled: **SAG RT or LT KIDNEY LONG AXIS and PERFUSION**

9. Doppler spectral waveforms from the renal medulla **(A)** and cortex **(B)**.

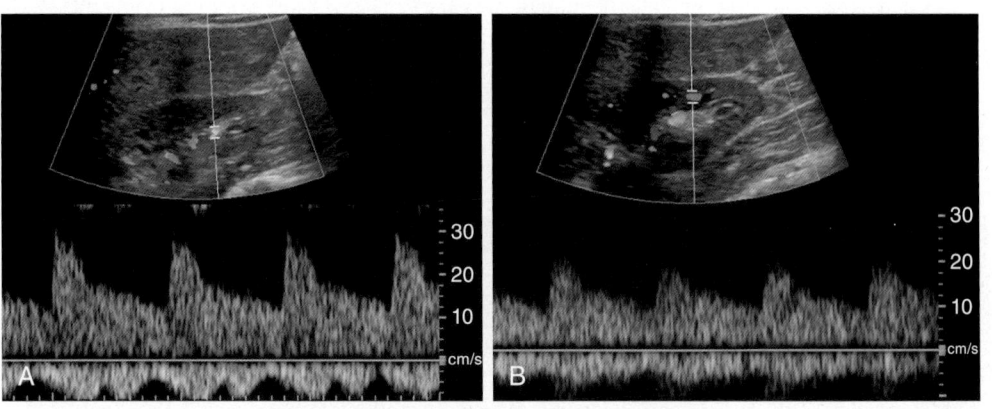

Labeled: **RT or LT REN MEDULLA/CORTEX**

SCANNING TIP: Approximately 20% of patients will have more than 1 renal artery on each side. For reasons that are not well understood, this finding is more commonly seen on the left side than on the right.

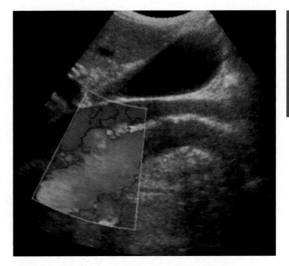

Examples of Various Venous Blood Flow Patterns and Duplex Protocols

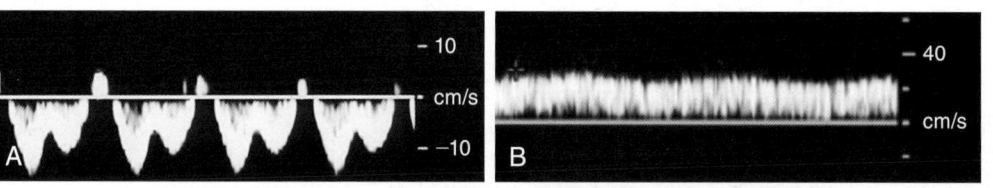

Venous Doppler spectral waveforms demonstrating the pulsatile flow
pattern found in a hepatic vein **(A)** and the minimally phasic flow
pattern found in the main portal vein **(B)**.

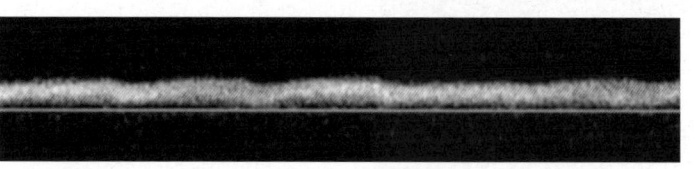

Gray-scale version of the color Doppler spectral waveform
demonstrating absence of respiratory phasicity.

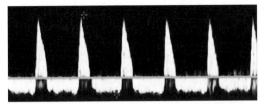

Doppler spectral waveforms recorded within the renal parenchyma demonstrating the blood flow pattern consistent with renal vein thrombosis.

Examples of Gynecological and Obstetric Doppler Spectral Waveforms

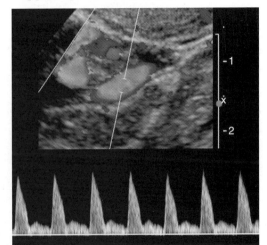

Gray-scale version of the color Doppler spectral waveforms from the uterine artery in a nongravid woman. (Courtesy Philips Medical Ultrasound, Seattle, Wash.)

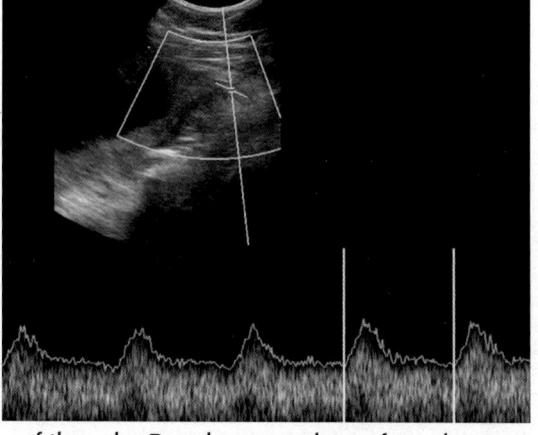

Gray-scale version of the color Doppler spectral waveform demonstrating absence of respiratory phasicity. (Courtesy Janice Hickey-Scharf, Picton, Ont., Canada.)

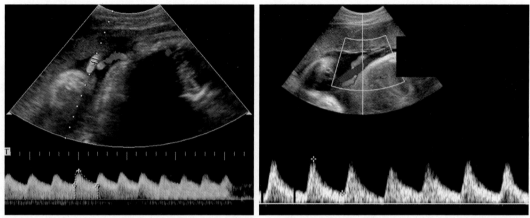

Gray-scale versions of the color Doppler spectral waveforms from umbilical arteries demonstrating variation in the level of vascular resistance. (Courtesy Janice Hickey-Scharf, Picton, Ont., Canada.)

Image Examples of Various Studies

Abdominal Venous Flow Study

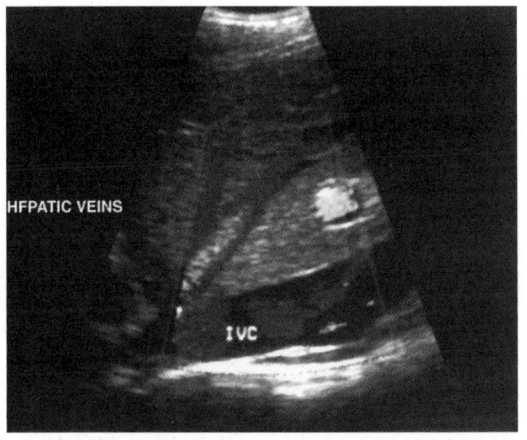

Gray-scale version of color flow Doppler in hepatic veins.

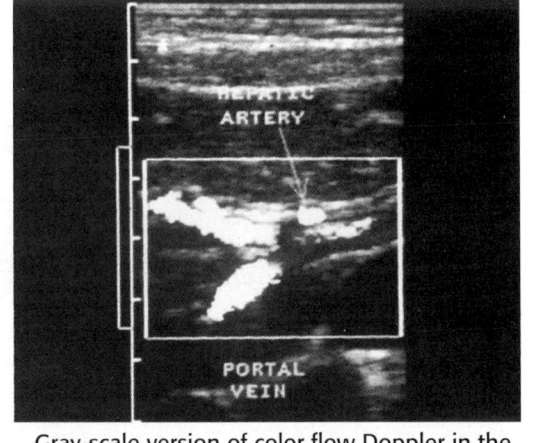

Gray-scale version of color flow Doppler in the portal vein.

Obstetrical Study

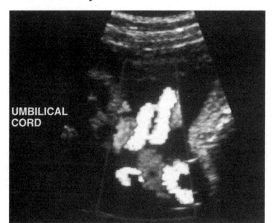

Gray-scale version of color Doppler in the 3-vessel umbilical cord.

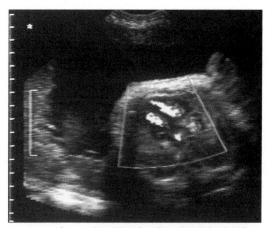

Gray-scale version of color flow Doppler in the 4-chamber fetal heart.

Gynecological Study

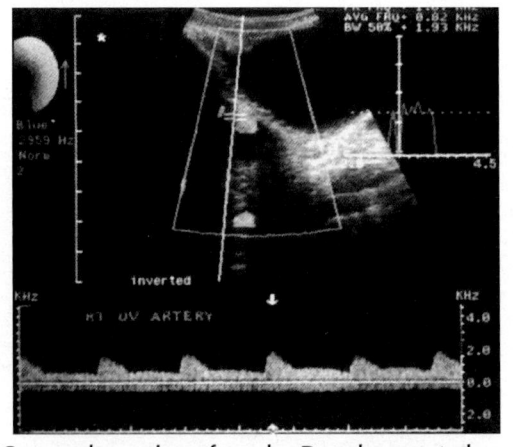

Gray-scale version of a color Doppler spectral display of blood in an active ovary.

Scrotal Study

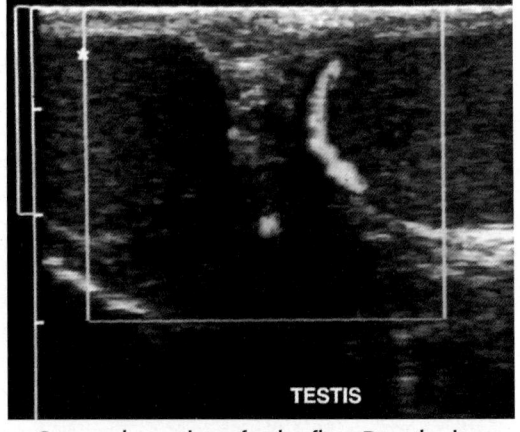

Gray-scale version of color flow Doppler in a testicular artery.

SECTION TWO ▪ Image Protocol for Cerebrovascular Duplex Scanning

Criteria

- Do not share the results of the study with the patient. Legally, only physicians can give a diagnosis.

Cerebrovascular Study

1. Longitudinal B-Mode image of the right proximal common carotid artery.

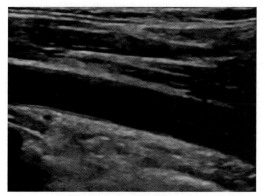

Labeled: **SAG RT PCCA**

2. Spectral waveforms from the right proximal common carotid artery *with peak systolic and end diastolic velocities measured.*

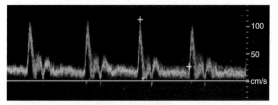

Labeled: **RT PCCA**

3. Longitudinal B-Mode image of the right middle common carotid artery.

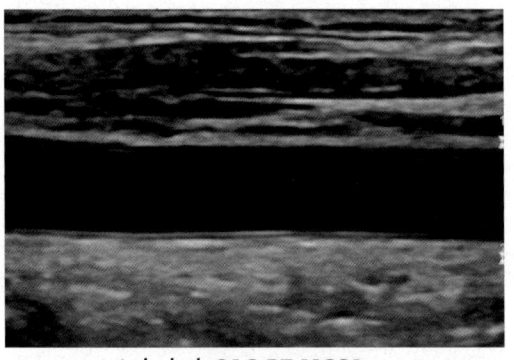

Labeled: **SAG RT MCCA**

4. Spectral waveforms from the right middle common carotid artery *with peak systolic and end diastolic velocities measured.*

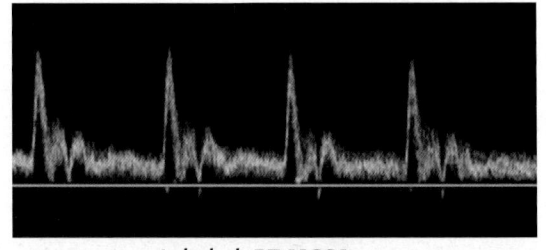

Labeled: **RT MCCA**

5. Longitudinal B-Mode image of the right distal common carotid artery.

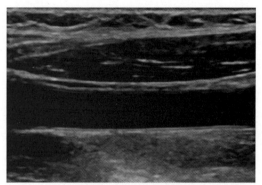

Labeled: **SAG RT DCCA**

6. Spectral waveforms from the right distal common carotid artery *with peak systolic and end diastolic velocities measured.*

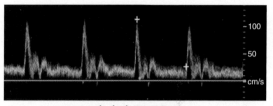

Labeled: **RT DCCA**

7. Longitudinal B-Mode image of the right carotid bulb (bifurcation).

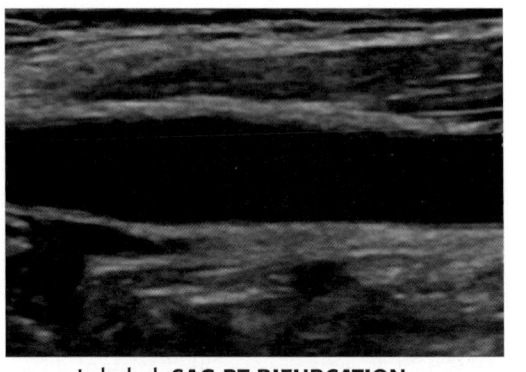

Labeled: **SAG RT BIFURCATION**

8. Spectral waveforms from the right carotid bulb *with peak systolic and end diastolic velocities measured.*

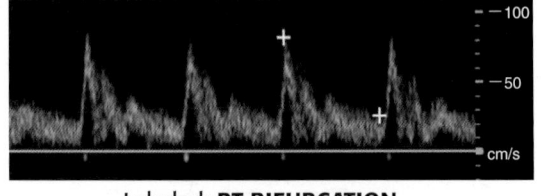

Labeled: **RT BIFURCATION**

9. Longitudinal B-Mode image of the right proximal internal carotid artery at its origin.

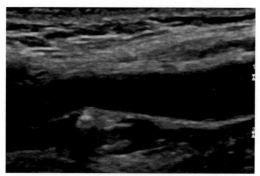

Labeled: **SAG RT PICA**

10. Spectral waveforms from the right proximal internal carotid artery *with peak and end diastolic velocities measured.*

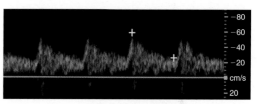

Labeled: **RT PICA**

11. Longitudinal B-Mode image of the right mid-segment of the internal carotid artery.

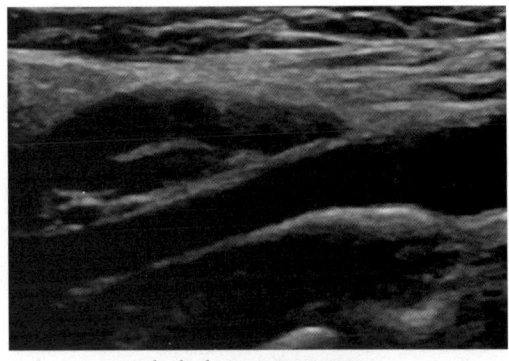

Labeled: **SAG RT MICA**

12. Spectral waveforms from the right mid segment of the internal carotid artery *with peak and end diastolic velocities measured.*

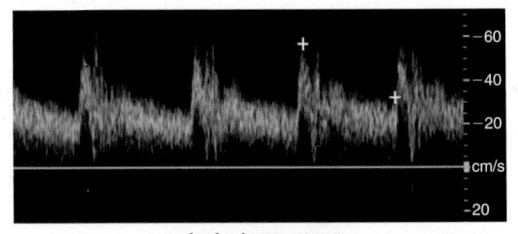

Labeled: **RT MICA**

13. Longitudinal B-Mode image of the right distal internal carotid artery.

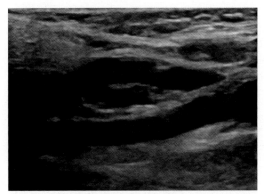

Labeled: **SAG RT DICA**

14. Spectral waveforms from the right distal internal carotid artery *with peak and end diastolic velocities measured.*

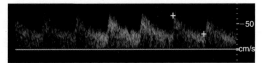

Labeled: **RT DICA**

15. Longitudinal B-Mode image of the right external carotid artery.

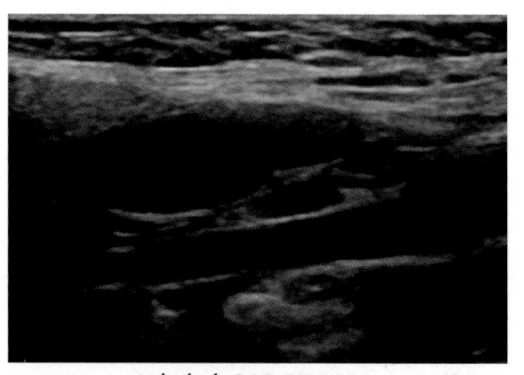

Labeled: **SAG RT ECA**

16. Spectral waveforms representing the right external carotid artery flow pattern *with peak and end diastolic velocities measured.*

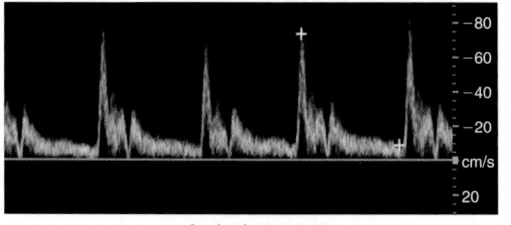

Labeled: **RT ECA**

17. Optional longitudinal B-Mode image of the right vertebral artery in the midcervical segment of the neck.

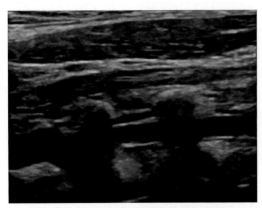

Labeled: **SAG MIDCERVICAL RT VERT**

18. Spectral waveforms from the right midcervical segment of the vertebral artery *with peak systolic and end diastolic velocities measured.*

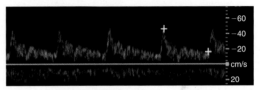

Labeled: **MIDCERVICAL RT VERT**

19. Longitudinal B-Mode image of the right vertebral artery at its origin from the right subclavian artery.

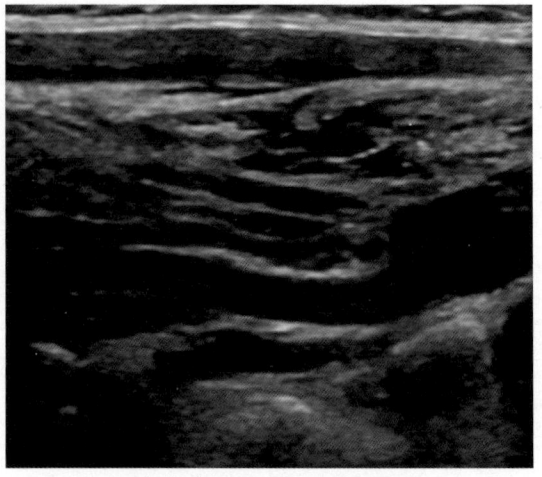

Labeled: **SAG PROX RT VERT**

20. Spectral waveforms from the right proximal vertebral artery *with peak systolic and end diastolic velocities measured.*

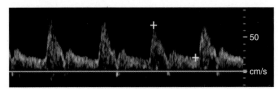

Labeled: **PROX RT VERT**

SCANNING TIP: Repeat the required images on the left side beginning with a thorough survey.

NOTE: Even in the absence of visible signs of pathology, it is important to carefully image the carotid bulb. It is thought that this area is most prone to atherosclerosis because of shear forces imposed on the arterial wall by the moving blood and by the geometry of this region of the bifurcation. Stenotic lesions often remain asymptomatic until they produce a pressure-flow gradient (reduce the diameter of the arterial lumen by more than 60%). Lesser lesions may be detected only with careful, thorough scanning in the transverse and longitudinal planes.

SECTION THREE ▪ Image Protocols for Peripheral Arterial and Venous Duplex Scanning

Criteria

- Do not share the results of the study with the patient. Legally, only physicians can give a diagnosis.

Lower Limb Arterial Duplex Study

1. Longitudinal image of the mid-to-distal abdominal aorta.

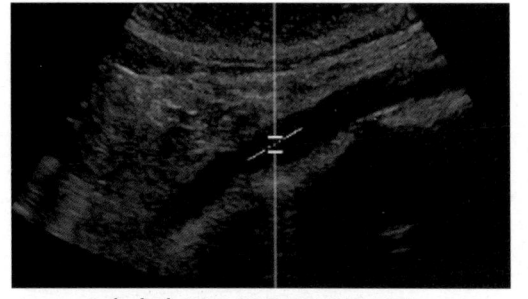

Labeled: **SAG MID-TO-DIST AO**

2. Doppler spectral waveform from the mid-to-distal abdominal aorta.

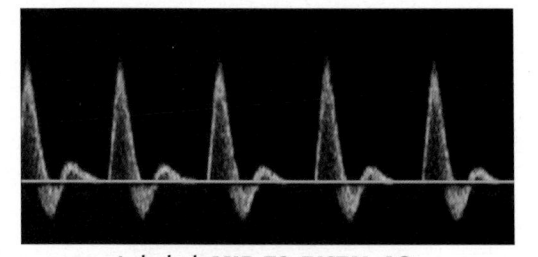

Labeled: **MID-TO-DISTAL AO**

3. Longitudinal image of the common iliac artery.

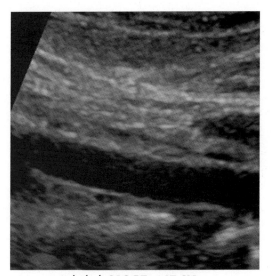

Labeled: **SAG RT or LT CIA**

4. Doppler spectral waveforms from the common iliac artery.

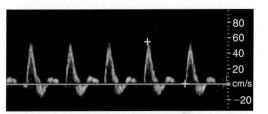

Labeled: **RT or LT CIA**

5. Longitudinal image of the external iliac artery.

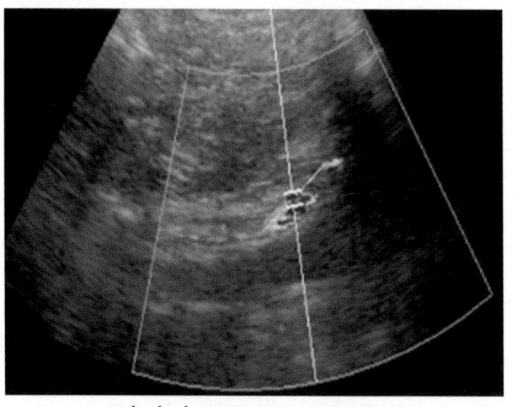

Labeled: **SAG RT or LT EIA**

6. Doppler spectral waveform from the external iliac artery.

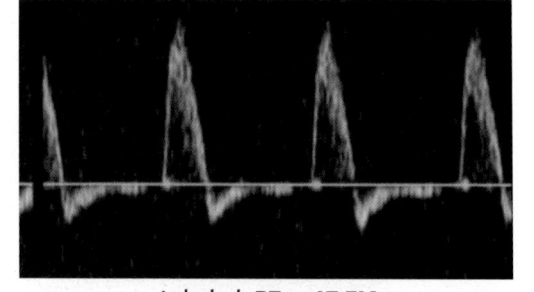

Labeled: **RT or LT EIA**

7. Longitudinal image of the common femoral artery.

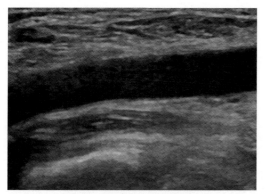

Labeled: **SAG RT or LT CFA**

8. Doppler spectral waveform from the common femoral artery.

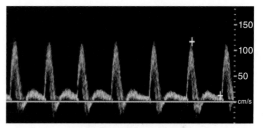

Labeled: **RT or LT CFA**

9. Longitudinal image of the proximal profunda femoris artery.

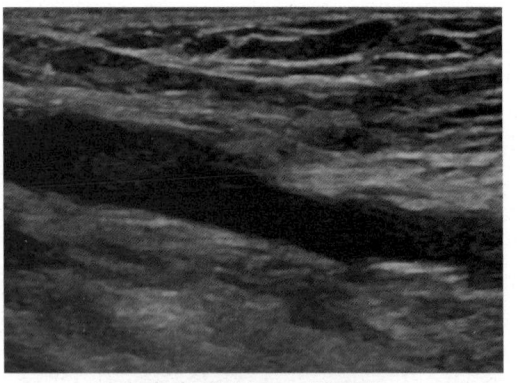

Labeled: **SAG RT or LT PFA**

10. Doppler spectral waveform from the proximal profunda femoris artery.

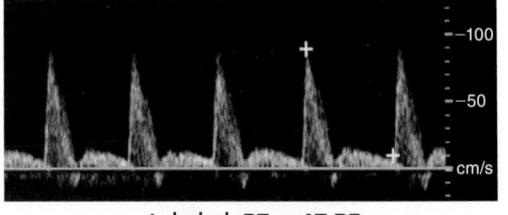

Labeled: **RT or LT PF**

11. Longitudinal image of the proximal superficial femoral artery.

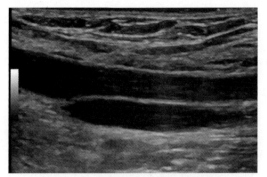

Labeled: **SAG RT or LT PROX SFA**

12. Doppler spectral waveform from the proximal superficial femoral artery.

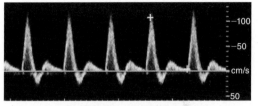

Labeled: **RT or LT PROX SFA**

Image Protocols for Peripheral Arterial and Venous Duplex Scanning ■ 487

13. Longitudinal image of the mid segment of the superficial femoral artery.

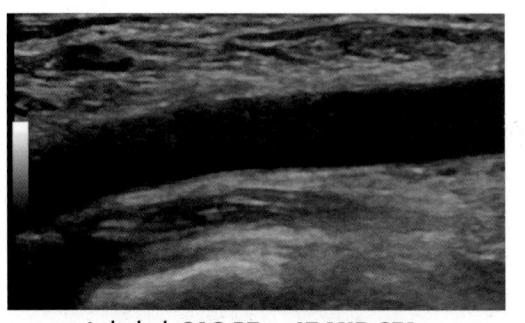

Labeled: **SAG RT or LT MID SFA**

14. Doppler spectral waveform from the mid segment of the superficial femoral artery.

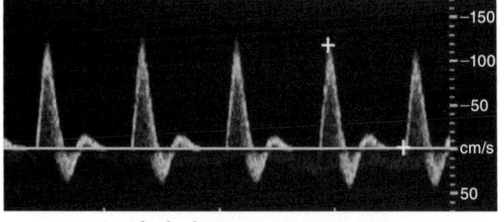

Labeled: **RT or LT MID SFA**

15. Longitudinal image of the distal superficial femoral artery.

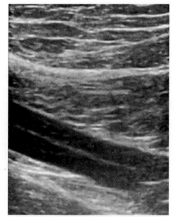

Labeled: **SAG RT or LT DIST SFA**

16. Doppler spectral waveform from the distal superficial femoral artery.

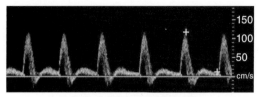

Labeled: **RT or LT DIST SFA**

17. Longitudinal image of the popliteal artery.

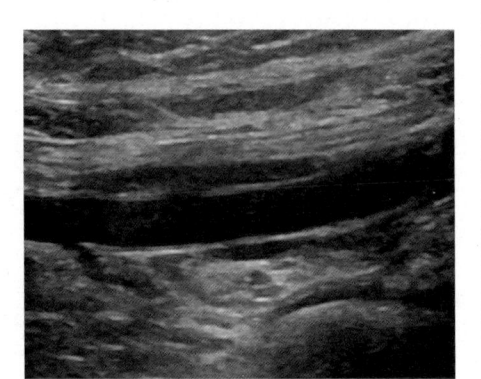

Labeled: **SAG RT or LT POP**

18. Doppler spectral waveform from the popliteal artery.

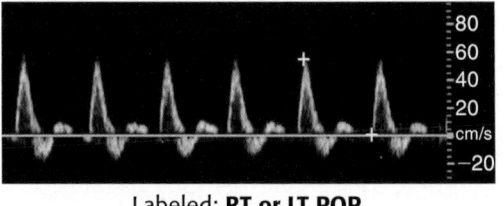

Labeled: **RT or LT POP**

19. Longitudinal image of the proximal anterior tibial artery.

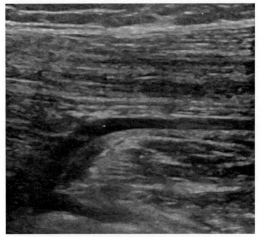

Labeled: **SAG RT or LT PROX AT**

20. Doppler spectral waveform from the proximal anterior tibial artery.

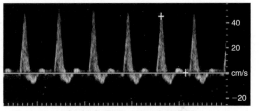

Labeled: **RT or LT PROX AT**

21. Longitudinal image of the proximal peroneal artery.

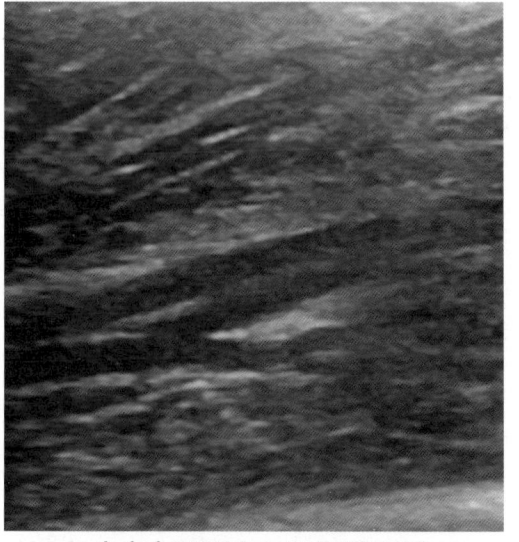

Labeled: **SAG RT or LT PROX PER**

22. Doppler spectral waveform from the proximal peroneal artery.

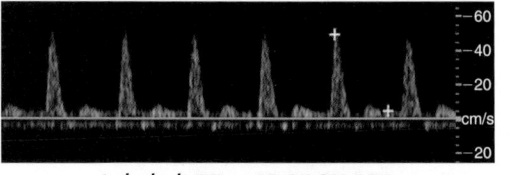

Labeled: **RT or LT PROX PER**

23. Longitudinal image of the mid segment of the peroneal artery.

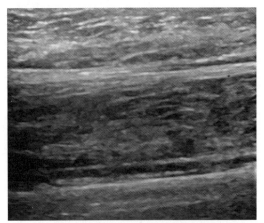

Labeled: **SAG RT or LT MID PER**

24. Doppler spectral waveform from the mid segment of the peroneal artery.

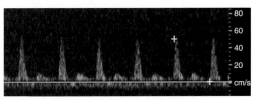

Labeled: **RT or LT MID PER**

25. Longitudinal image of the distal peroneal artery.

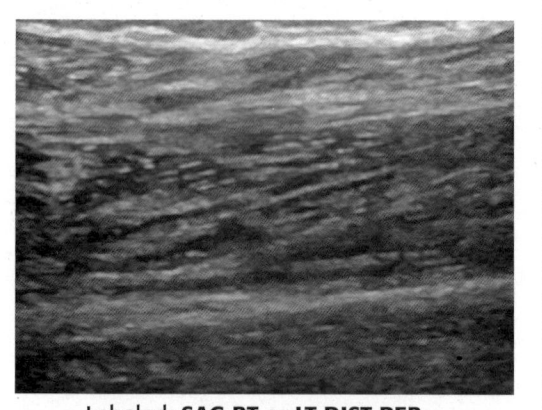

Labeled: **SAG RT or LT DIST PER**

26. Doppler spectral waveform from the distal peroneal artery.

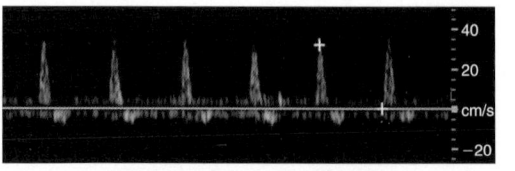

Labeled: **RT or LT DIST PER**

27. Longitudinal image of the proximal posterior tibial artery.

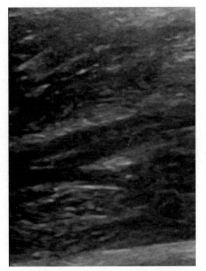

Labeled: **SAG RT or LT PROX PT**

28. Doppler spectral waveform from the proximal posterior tibial artery.

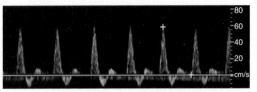

Labeled: **RT or LT PROX PT**

29. Longitudinal image of the mid segment of the posterior tibial artery.

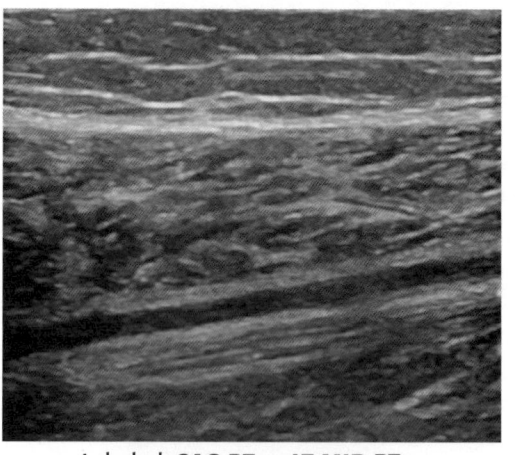

Labeled: **SAG RT or LT MID PT**

30. Doppler spectral waveform from the mid segment of the posterior tibial artery.

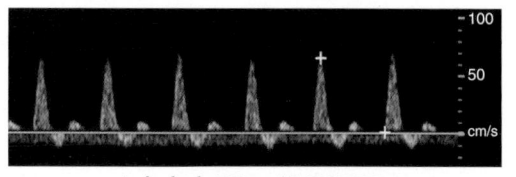

Labeled: **RT or LT MID PT**

31. Longitudinal image of the distal posterior tibial artery.

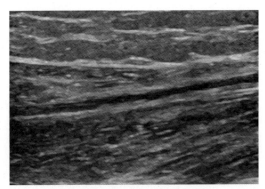

Labeled: **SAG RT or LT DIST PT**

32. Doppler spectral waveform from the distal posterior tibial artery.

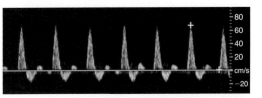

Labeled: **RT or LT DIST PT**

Lower Limb Venous Duplex Study

1. Split-screen axial images of noncompressed and compressed common femoral vein.

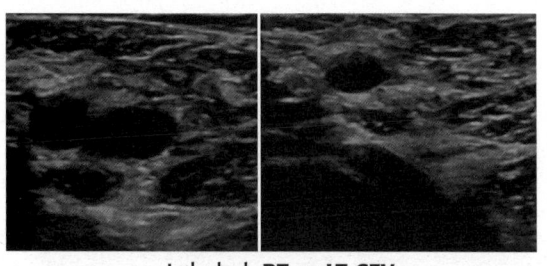

Labeled: **RT or LT CFV**

2. Doppler spectral waveforms from the common femoral vein.

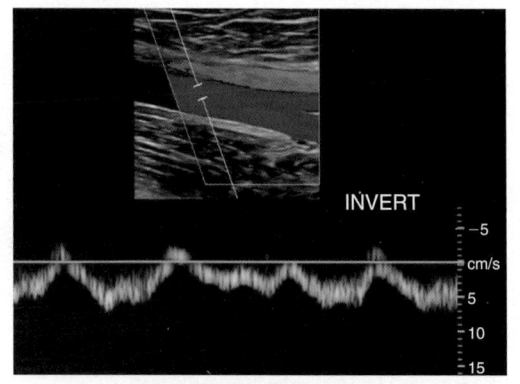

Labeled: **RT or LT CFV**
Gray-scale version. See Color Plate 29
in *Sonography Scanning.*

3. Split-screen axial images of noncompressed and compressed profunda femoris vein.

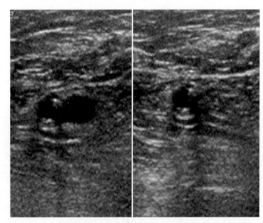

Labeled: **RT or LT PFV**

4. Doppler spectral waveforms from the profunda femoris vein.

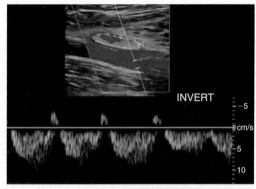

Labeled: **RT or LT PFV**

5. Split-screen axial images of noncompressed and compressed proximal, mid, and distal femoral vein.

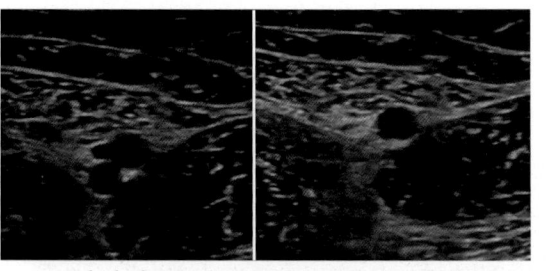

Labeled: **RT or LT PROX, MID, or DIST FV**

6. Doppler spectral waveforms from the proximal, mid, and distal femoral vein.

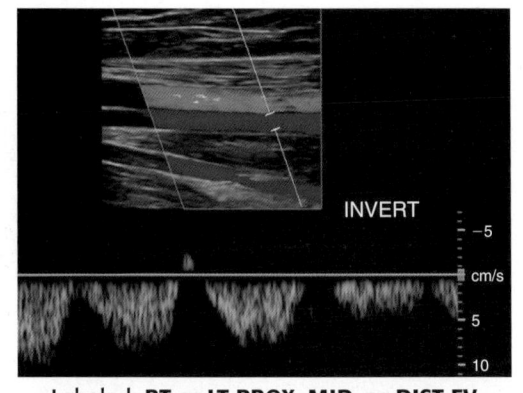

Labeled: **RT or LT PROX, MID, or DIST FV**

7. Split-screen axial images of noncompressed and compressed popliteal vein.

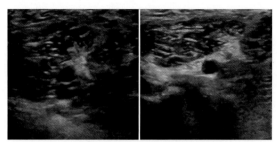

Labeled: **RT or LT POPLITEAL V**

8. Doppler spectral waveforms from the popliteal vein.

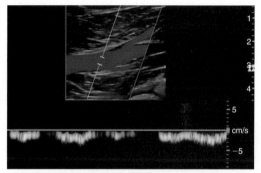

Labeled: **RT or LT POPLITEAL V**

9. Split-screen images of noncompressed and compressed gastrocnemius veins.

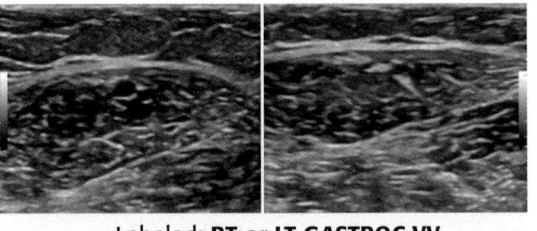

Labeled: **RT or LT GASTROC VV**

10. Split-screen axial images of noncompressed and compressed proximal anterior tibial veins.

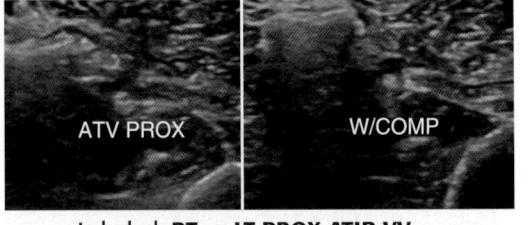

Labeled: **RT or LT PROX ATIB VV**

11. Split-screen axial images of noncompressed and compressed tibioperoneal trunk.

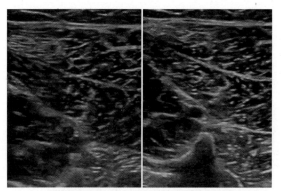

Labeled: **RT or LT TIBPER TRUNK**

12. Split-screen axial images of noncompressed and compressed proximal, mid, and distal peroneal veins.

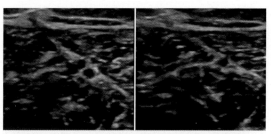

Labeled: **RT or LT PROX, MID, or DIST PER VV**

13. Doppler spectral waveforms from the proximal, mid, and distal peroneal veins (gray-scale version).

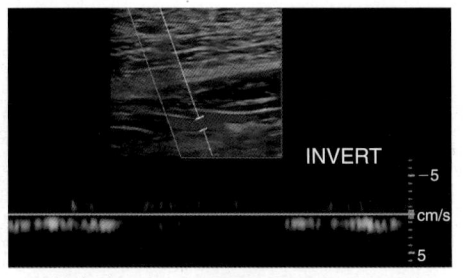

INVERT

Labeled: **RT or LT PROX, MID, or DIST PER VV**

14. Split-screen axial images of noncompressed and compressed proximal, mid, and distal posterior tibial veins.

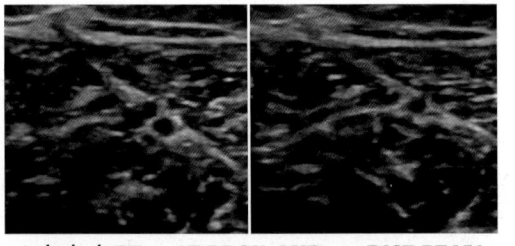

Labeled: **RT or LT PROX, MID, or DIST PT VV**

15. Doppler spectral waveforms from the proximal, mid, and distal posterior tibial veins (gray-scale version).

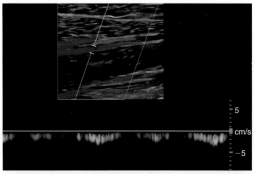

Labeled: **RT or LT PROX, MID, or DIST PT VV**

16. Split-screen axial images of noncompressed and compressed proximal, mid, and distal small saphenous vein.

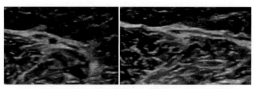

Labeled: **RT or LT PROX, MID, or DIST SSV**

17. Doppler spectral waveforms from the proximal, mid, and distal small saphenous vein (gray-scale version).

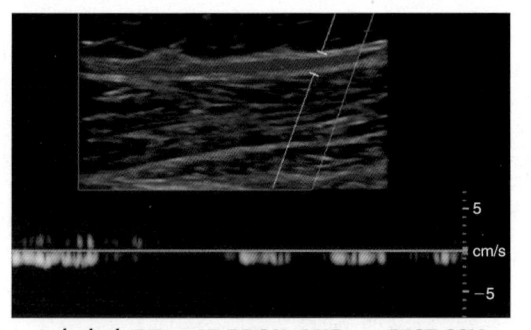

Labeled: **RT or LT PROX, MID, or DIST SSV**

18. Split-screen axial images of noncompressed and compressed proximal, mid, and distal thigh segments of the great saphenous vein.

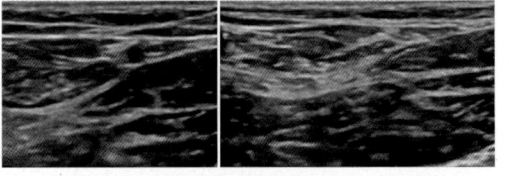

Labeled: **RT or LT PROX, MID, or DIST THIGH GSV**

19. Doppler spectral waveforms from the proximal, mid, and distal thigh and calf segments and at the knee of the great saphenous vein (gray-scale version).

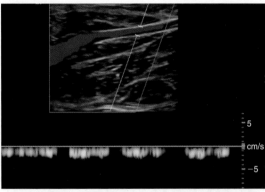

Labeled: **RT** or **LT PROX, MID,** or **DIST THIGH GSV**

ECHOCARDIOGRAPHY

SECTION ONE ▪ Image Protocol for the Sonographic Study of the Adult Heart

Adult Heart Study

SCANNING TIP: The study is videotaped allowing for real-time assessment of structures. At least 6 to 10 beats of each view should be recorded with additional images of any pathology.

SCANNING TIP: The anterior portion of the aortic root and the interventricular septum should be continuous and as perpendicular to the ultrasound beam as possible. The posterior portion of the aortic root runs continuous with the anterior mitral valve leaflet.

1. Parasternal long axis.

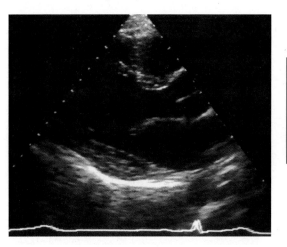

2. Right ventricular inflow view.

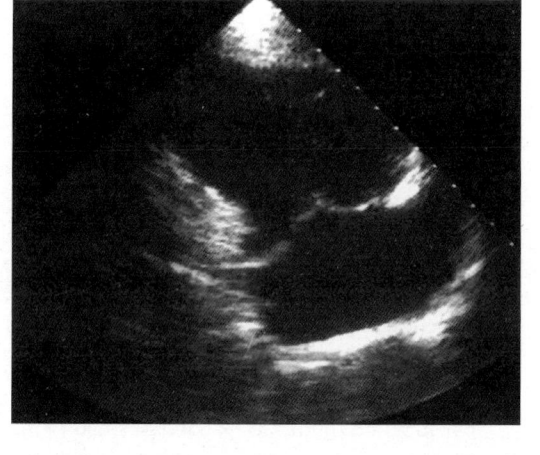

3. Right ventricular outflow view.

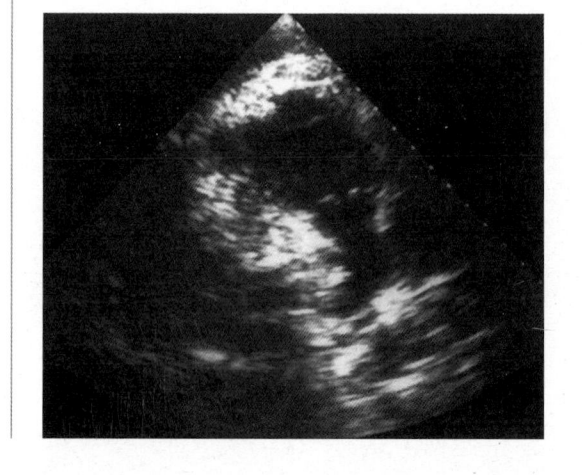

4. Parasternal short axis at the level of the aortic valve.

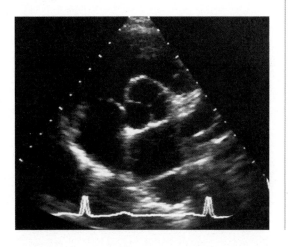

5. Parasternal short axis at the level of the mitral valve.

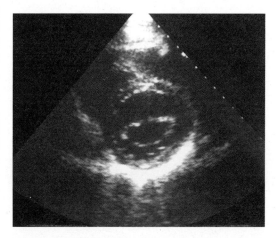

6. Parasternal short axis at the level of the papillary muscles.

7. Apical 4-chamber view.

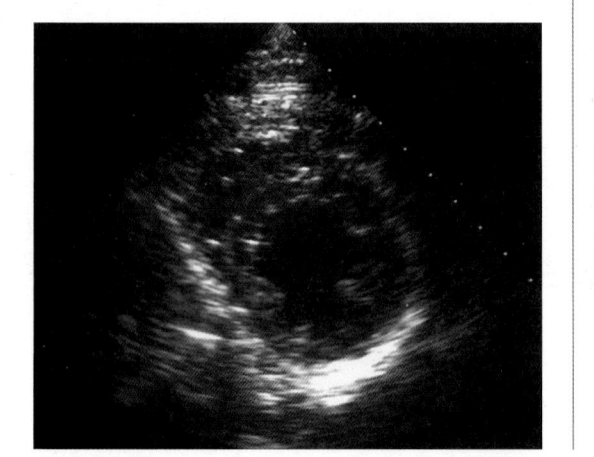

8. Apical 5-chamber view.

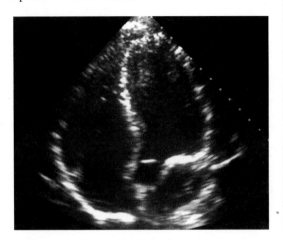

9. Apical 2-chamber view.

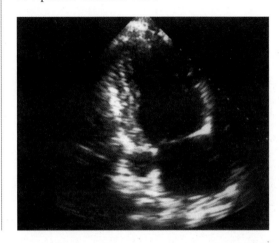

SCANNING TIP: When questions involving the aorta arise, a portion of the descending thoracic aorta can be visualized posterior to the 2-chamber view and should be evaluated for pathology.

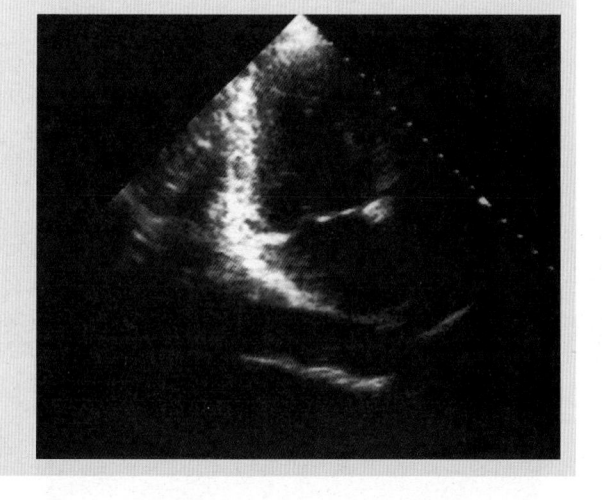

10. Apical long axis.

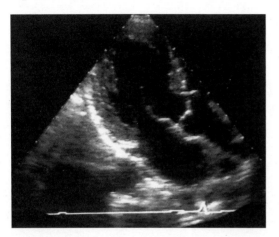

11. Subxiphoid 4-chamber view.

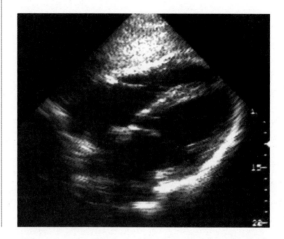

12. Subxiphoid short axis papillary muscle level.

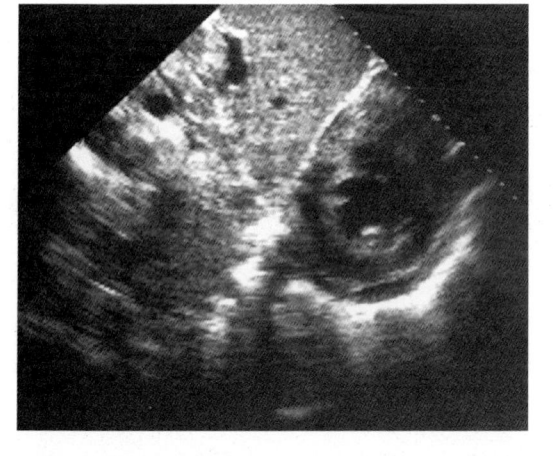

13. Subxiphoid short axis at the level of the mitral valve.

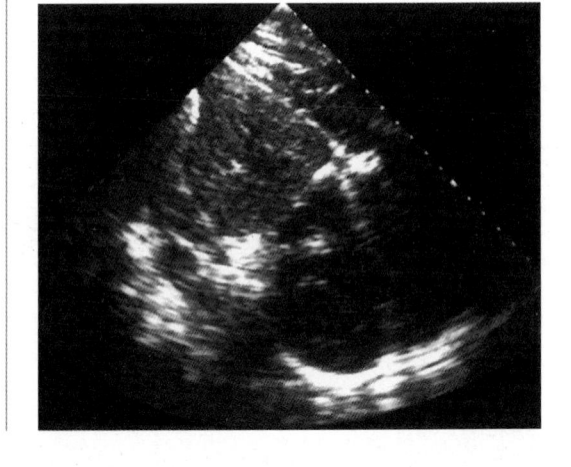

14. Subxiphoid short axis at the level of the aortic valve.

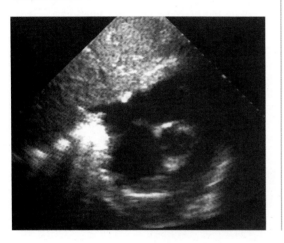

15. Subxiphoid short axis viewing the IVC entering the RA.

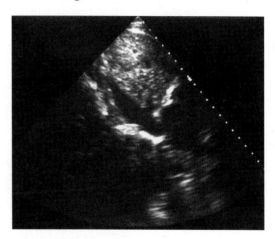

16. Suprasternal notch viewing the long axis of the aorta.

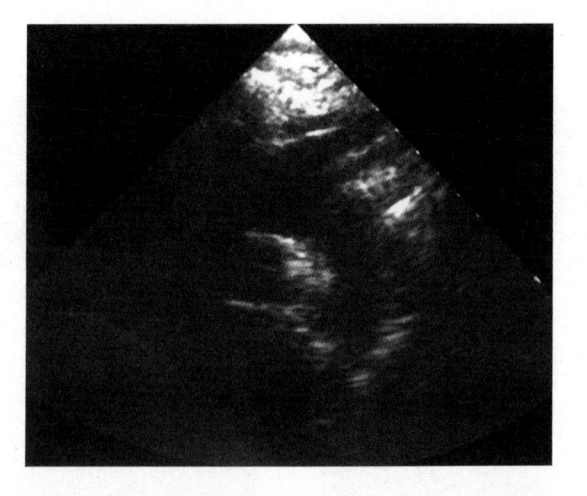

SCANNING TIP: This view should be used when questions involving the aorta arise, such as dissection or Marfan syndrome. A short axis of the aorta should also be evaluated in these cases.

M-Mode Evaluation

The M-Mode is a 2-dimensional graphic drawing of the heart used to measure distance over time. An M-Mode is useful for obtaining dimensions of the heart and assessing fine movements too subtle for the eye to see.

SCANNING TIP: A minimum of 6 beats should be recorded at each level demonstrating both systolic and diastolic motion.

SCANNING TIP: The M-Mode may be documented on either videotape or strip chart recorder. If the strip chart is used, begin with a frozen image of the parasternal long axis view to demonstrate the orientation of the heart.

SCANNING TIP: The 2-D image must be as perpendicular to the ultrasound beam as possible, lessening the chance for inaccurate measurements. (A tipped ventricle will yield exaggerated numbers.) When measuring, if unsure of a dimension, omit it.

Aortic Valve Level

- The cursor is placed so that it transects the RV, aorta, and LA in either the parasternal long or short axis view.

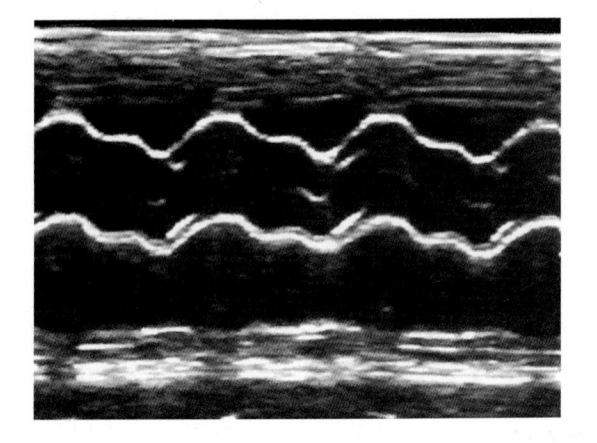

- Measurements taken:*
  1. *Aortic root:* from the anterior wall of the root to the posterior wall of the root, at the level of the Q wave on the ECG; normally 1.9 to 4 cm.
  2. *Aortic valve cusp separation:* normally has the shape of a box when open with the right coronary cusp more anterior and the noncoronary cusp posterior. Measured at the onset of systole (when the valve first opens); normally 1.5 to 2.6 cm.
  3. *Left atrium:* measured at the largest dimension (end systole); normally 1.9 to 4 cm.

SCANNING TIP: Always measure structures from leading edge to leading edge.

Aortic root dimension   Aortic cusp separation   Left atrial dimension

*Normal values used in the laboratory at Thomas Jefferson University, Philadelphia, Pa.

PART VIII

Mitral Valve Level

- Slowly sweep the cursor through the LVOT region to the tip of the mitral valve leaflets. This sweep will demonstrate structural continuity. The biphasic opening of both mitral leaflets should then be documented.

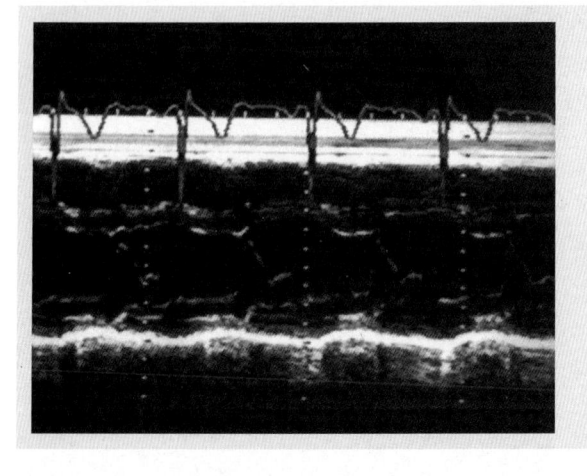

SCANNING TIP: The mitral valve is labeled to describe the different phases of its motion.

D: Beginning of diastole
E: Maximal excursion of the valve
F: Point to which the valve had closed following the passive filling phase
A: Atrial contraction (P wave on the ECG)
B: Extra bump between A and C (occurs only when pathology, such as diastolic dysfunction, is present)
C: Closure of the valve and the beginning of systole

- Measurements:*
  1. D to E excursion; normally greater than 1.6 cm.
  2. E to F slope over the period of 1 second (expressed in mm/sec); normally greater than 70 mm/sec.
  3. E point to septal separation; normally no greater than 1 cm.

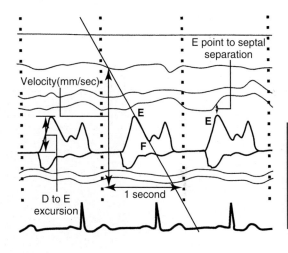

*Normal values used in the laboratory at Thomas Jefferson University, Philadelphia, Pa.

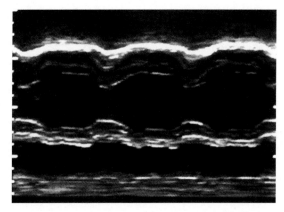

Left Ventricular Level

Slowly sweep the cursor just beyond the mitral leaflets but stop before the papillary muscles. Both systolic and diastolic dimensions of the LV should be documented.

- Measurements:*
  1. All of the following are measured at the level of the Q wave on the ECG: RV (no greater than 2.7 cm); IVS, posterior LV wall (both normally between 0.6 and 1.2 cm); and LV end diastolic dimension (LVEDD) (normal range 3.5 to 5.7 cm).

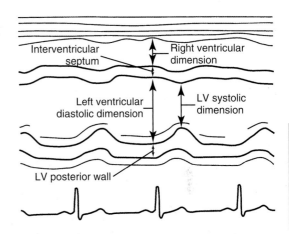

PART VIII

SCANNING TIP: Often the free wall of the RV is not visualized because of its close proximity to the transducer, making it difficult to determine the true size of the chamber. The measurement is therefore taken from the point where motion is first observed, to the leading edge of the interventricular septum. Then subtract 0.5 cm from the total to compensate for the RV wall thickness.

2. LV end systolic dimension (LVESD): measure at the smallest dimension.

SCANNING TIP: The LVEDD and the LVESD should be measured on the same beat.

SCANNING TIP: Be careful not to include chordae tendineae in the thickness of the LV walls.

Tricuspid and Pulmonic Valves

An M-Mode of the tricuspid or pulmonic valve is used to demonstrate thickness and motion and are not necessarily a routine part of the examination. There are no standard measurements obtained.

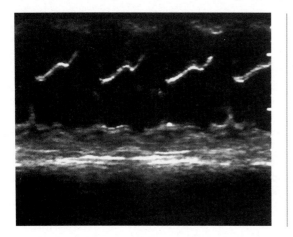
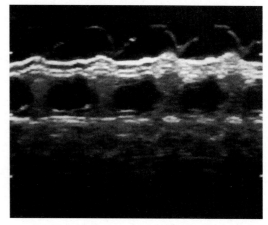

PART VIII

Doppler Evaluation

- Used to assess blood flow through the heart, including increased velocities, stenosis, regurgitation, and shunts.
- Continuous-wave (CW) and pulsed-wave (PW) Doppler are used in conjunction with each other. In addition, color Doppler simplifies the mapping process and gives a visual representation of the size and direction of blood flow disturbances.

Normal Valve Profiles
Mitral Valve

- The flow profile is shaped like an M and is best sampled in the apical 4-chamber view. Here, blood flow moves towards the transducer during diastole; therefore the waveform appears above the baseline. Peak velocity should not exceed 1.3 m/sec.*

---

*Hatle L, Angelsen B: *Doppler ultrasound in cardiology,* ed. 2, Philadelphia, 1985, Lea & Febiger, p. 93.

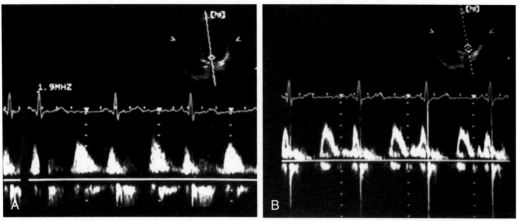

A, Continuous-wave mitral valve Doppler. **B,** Pulsed-wave mitral valve Doppler.

SCANNING TIP: PW Doppler has an envelope (whiter outline) and window (darker interior) versus the filled-in profile of continuous-wave Doppler. In cases of turbulent flow, this PW window can become filled in and is called spectral broadening.

Tricuspid Valve

- The flow profile also looks like an M and occurs during diastole. It is best sampled in either the right ventricular inflow view or the apical 4-chamber view. Blood flow moves towards the transducer; therefore, the profile appears above the baseline. Peak velocity should not exceed 0.7 m/sec.*

---

*Hatle L, Angelsen B: *Doppler ultrasound in cardiology,* ed. 2, Philadelphia, 1985, Lea & Febiger, p. 93.

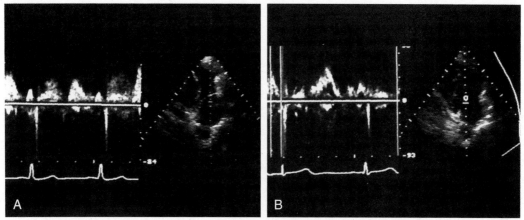

A, Continuous-wave tricuspid valve Doppler. **B,** Pulsed-wave tricuspid valve Doppler.

Aortic Valve

- A sample is best taken from the apical 5-chamber view and the profile has the shape of a bullet. In this case, blood flow is moving away from the transducer during systole and therefore appears below the baseline. Peak velocity should not exceed 1.7 m/sec.*

*Hatle L, Angelsen B: *Doppler ultrasound in cardiology,* ed. 2, Philadelphia, 1985, Lea & Febiger, p. 93.

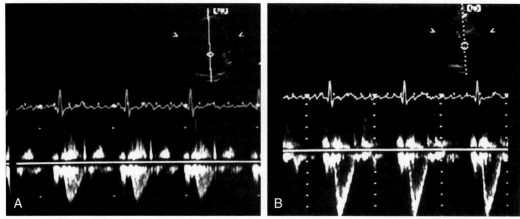

A, Continuous-wave aortic valve Doppler. **B,** Pulsed-wave aortic valve Doppler.

Pulmonic Valve

- The profile is also shaped like a bullet, but is best sampled in parasternal short axis at the level of the aortic valve. Flow moves away from the transducer during systole; therefore it appears below the baseline. Peak velocity should not exceed 0.9 m/sec.*

---

*Hatle L, Angelsen B: *Doppler ultrasound in cardiology,* ed. 2, Philadelphia, 1985, Lea & Febiger, p. 93.

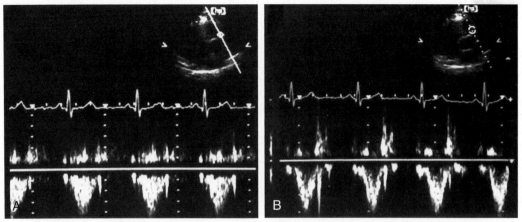

A, Continuous-wave pulmonic valve Doppler. **B,** Pulsed-wave pulmonic valve Doppler.

Left Ventricular Outflow Tract

- Systolic flow sampled in this region is also shaped like a bullet and appears below the baseline. It is best sampled in the apical 5-chamber view and peak velocity should not exceed 1.1 m/sec.*

SCANNING TIP: Doppler is best when flow is parallel to the ultrasound beam. In contrast, 2-D is best when perpendicular. Therefore, the best Doppler image is not necessarily the best 2-D image.

Valve Survey

SCANNING TIP: The following sequence should be used in the evaluation of each valve: color Doppler, continuous-wave (CW) Doppler, then PW Doppler. Assess each value separately beginning with the mitral valve. Repeat this process on the aortic, tricuspid, and pulmonic valves, and the left ventricular outflow tract (LVOT) if necessary.

---

*Hatle L, Angelsen B: *Doppler ultrasound in cardiology,* ed. 2, Philadelphia, 1985, Lea & Febiger, p. 93.

Color Doppler Survey

> **SCANNING TIP:** Flow moving towards the transducer appears as various shades of red. Flow moving away is blue. A lower velocity would be deeper in color and gradually lighten as the velocity increases to almost yellow or white. At times, a variance map is used. This is usually a green color tagged on the end of the color spectrum. The green makes the higher velocities or turbulent flows stand out.
>
> **SCANNING TIP:** Regurgitation or any pathology should be demonstrated in more than 1 view.

- The color sector should be placed so that the valve or area being assessed is in the center of the sample. Normally, mitral and tricuspid flow appear red, and pulmonic and aortic flow are blue. When the valves are closed, no color (regurgitation) should be seen below them. Mitral and tricuspid regurgitation appear blue; aortic and pulmonic regurgitation are usually red.
- Slowly angle the transducer back and forth across the valve plane to locate any eccentric areas of turbulence. Demonstrate the size and location of any regurgitation or turbulent flow.
- Color can also be used to locate the peak flow velocity across the valve allowing for easy placement of the CW Doppler cursor.

PART VIII

CW Doppler Survey

- CW is best for determining peak flow velocities. Place the cursor so it bisects the opening of the valve to be sampled. If the peak velocity across a valve exceeds its normal velocity, the peak should then be measured. Three profiles are measured and averaged. Do not measure post-PVC beats. If the patient is in atrial fibrillation, average at least 5 or 6 beats.
- The peak velocity of tricuspid regurgitation is also measured to help with the evaluation of pulmonary hypertension.

SCANNING TIP: If unable to find a peak velocity on any valve, tricuspid or aortic regurgitation, a nonimaging, stand-alone CW probe should be used. The peak velocity can be easily found because of the smaller footprint of the transducer and the lower frequency.

PW Doppler Survey

- PW Doppler demonstrates exactly where a flow disturbance occurs and is then used to map out the direction and size of the disturbance. Place the cursor or Doppler "gate" slightly above the valve opening. Slowly move below the valve, then across the valve plane in both directions. If regurgitation is detected, follow the flow into the chamber as far back as it goes, mapping the length and also the width of the turbulent area.

SCANNING TIP: If any additional flow disturbances (e.g., ASD, VSD) are visualized, they too should be evaluated with color, PW, and CW Doppler.

SECTION TWO ■ Image Protocol for the Sonographic Study of the Pediatric Heart

Pediatric Heart Study

1. Subcostal view demonstrating the orientation of the aorta and IVC.

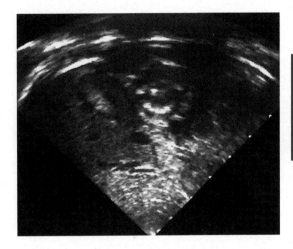

PART VIII

2. Subcostal 4-chamber view.

3. Subcostal 5-chamber view showing the aorta and the left ventricular outflow tract.

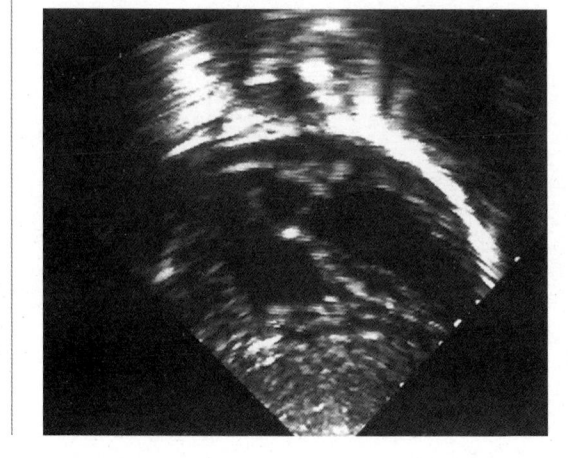

4. Subcostal long axis angled anteriorly to demonstrate the RV outflow tract, pulmonic valve, and the pulmonary artery.

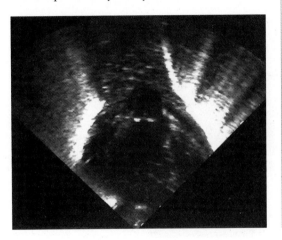

5. Short axis subcostal showing the IVC and SVC entering the right atrium.

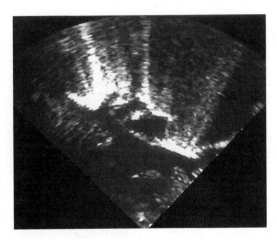

6. Short axis subcostal demonstrating the aortic valve, pulmonary artery, and interatrial septum.

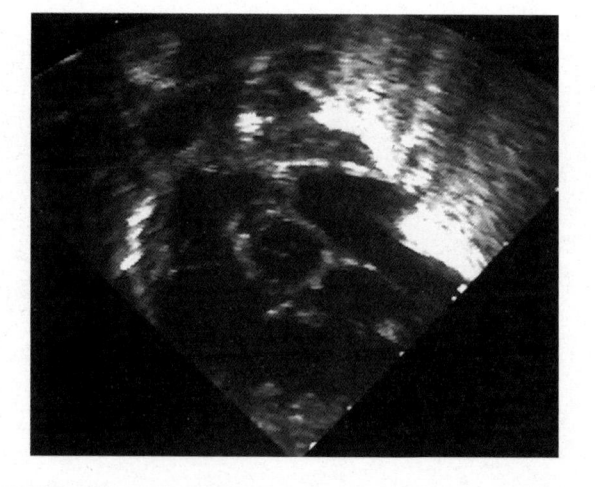

SCANNING TIP: A small angulation may be needed to fully visualize the interatrial septum.

7. Short axis subcostal of the mitral valve.

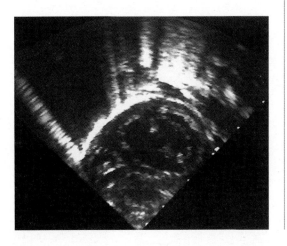

8. Short axis subcostal of the left and right ventricles.

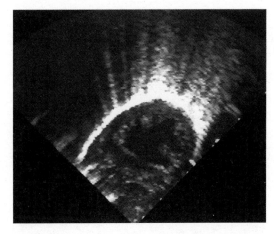

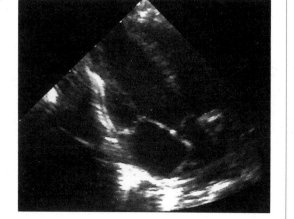

9. Apical 4-chamber view.

10. Apical long axis documenting the left ventricular outflow tract.

11. Parasternal long axis.

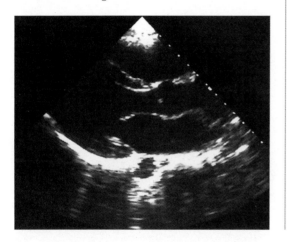

12. Right ventricular inflow view.

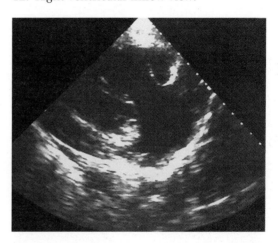

13. Right ventricular outflow view.

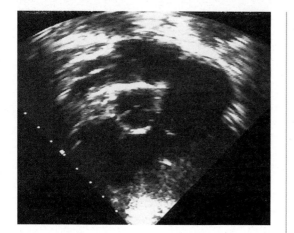

14. Parasternal short axis at the level of the aortic valve to document the orientation of the great vessels.

15. Parasternal short axis documenting the left coronary artery.

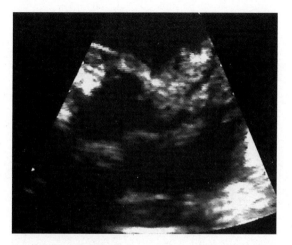

SCANNING TIP: Angle slightly above the aortic valve leaflets and zoom in on the region to simplify coronary evaluation.

16. Parasternal short axis documenting the right coronary artery.

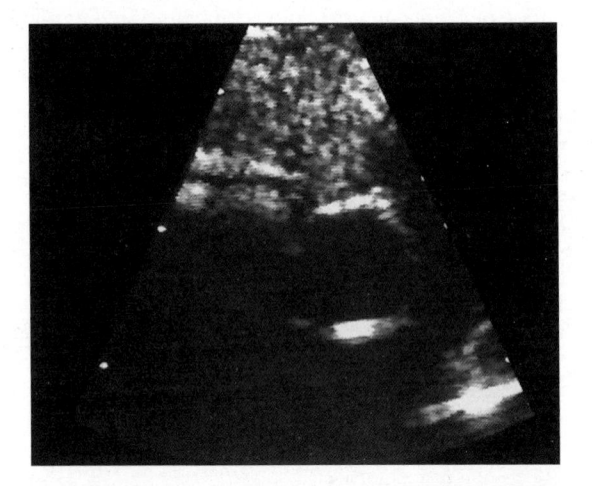

17. Parasternal short axis to document the right and left pulmonary branches and the presence/absence of a patent ductus arteriosus.

SCANNING TIP: If a ductus is present, demonstrate its connection to the aorta.

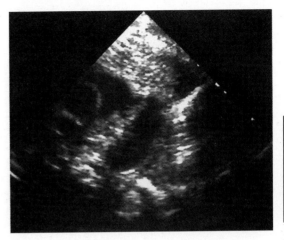

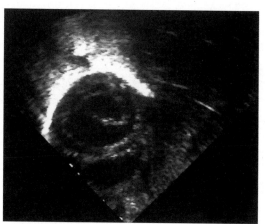

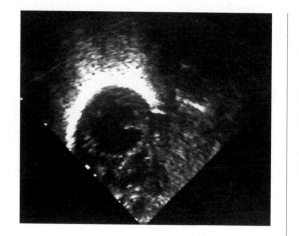

18. Parasternal short axis at the level of the mitral valve to document thickness and motion of the leaflets.

19. Parasternal short axis at the level of the papillary muscles.

20. Suprasternal notch documenting the aortic arch and its branches.

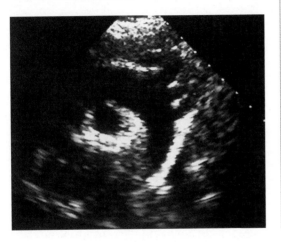

21. Suprasternal notch documenting the branch pulmonary arteries and short axis of the aorta.

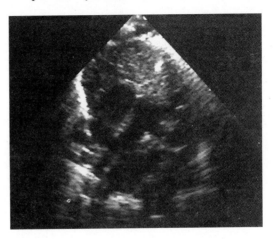

M-Mode evaluation

An M-Mode should be performed from either the parasternal long or the parasternal short axis by placing the cursor through the following 3 levels:

1. Aortic valve level

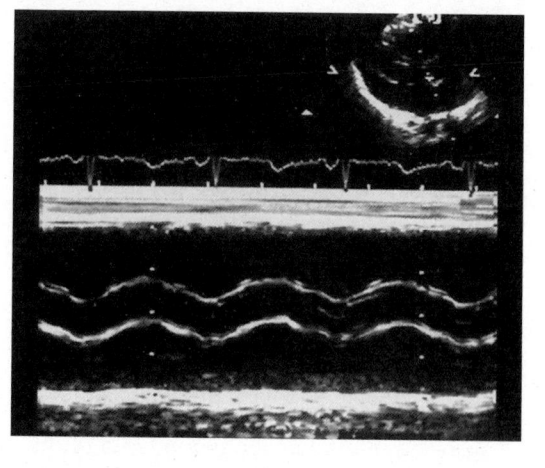

2. Mitral valve level

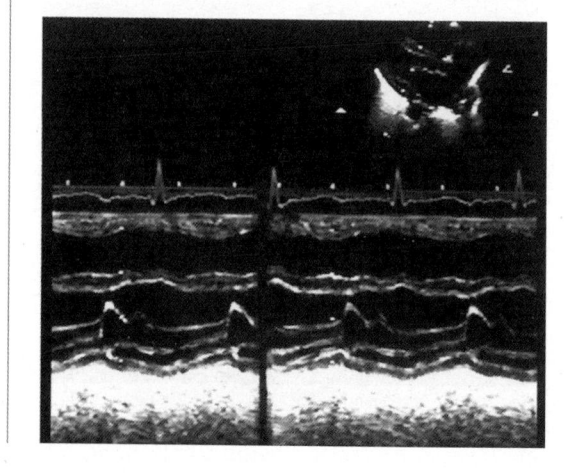

3. Left ventricular level.

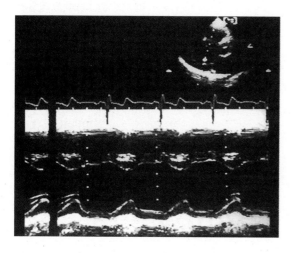

Attention is given to sizes of the chambers, motion of the valves, ventricular contractility, and structural continuity.

SCANNING TIP: Sweep speed of the M-Mode is increased to 100% to accommodate the increased heart rate of neonates.

ABBREVIATION GLOSSARY

AIUM: American Institute of Ultrasound in Medicine
ALARA: As low as reasonably acceptable
ANT: Anterior
ART: Artery
AV: Atrioventricular
AV: Atrioventricular valves
BIF: Bifurcation
CBD: Common bile duct
cc: Cubic centimeter
CD: Common duct
CERX: Cervix
CFA: Common femoral artery
CFV: Common femoral vein

CHD: Common hepatic duct
cm: Centimeter
COR: Coronal
CRL: Crown rump length
C-SPINE: Cervical spine
CW: Continuous-wave Doppler
DECUB: Decubitus
DP: Dorsalis pedis artery
ECG/EKG: Electrocardiogram
ER: Endorectal
EV: Endovaginal
Fd: Doppler shift frequency
Fo: Operating frequency
GB: Gallbladder

GS: Gestational sac
Hz: Hertz
IN: Inches
INF: Inferior
IVC: Inferior vena cava
IVS: Interventricular septum
kHz: Kilohertz
KID: Kidney
LA: Left atrium
LAD: Left anterior descending
LAT: Lateral
LLD: Left lateral decubitus
LPO: Left posterior oblique
L-SPINE: Lumbar spine
LT: Left
LV: Left ventricular
LVOT: Left ventricular outflow tract
MED: Medical
MHz: Megahertz
ML: Midline
mm: Millimeter
MV: Mitral valve

NIP: Nipple
OBL: Oblique
OV: Ovary
PA: Pulmonary artery
PDA: Patent ductus arteriosus
PFV: Profunda femoris vein
POP: Popliteal artery
POST: Posterior
PRF: Time and depth limitations
PROX: Proximal
PT: Posterior tibial artery
PV: Pulmonic valve
PW: Pulsed-wave Doppler
RA: Right atrium
RCA: Right coronary artery
RI: Resistive indices
RLD: Right lateral decubitus
RPO: Right posterior oblique
RT: Right
RV: Right ventricle
SA: Sinoatrial node
SAG: Sagittal

SEM V: Seminal vesicles
SFA: Superficial femoral artery
SFV: Superficial femoral vein
SMA: Superior mesenteric artery
SUP: Superior
SVC: Superior vena cava

TGC: Time-gain compensation
TRV: Transverse
T-SPINE: Thoracic spine
TV: Tricuspid valve
UT: Uterus
VAG: Vagina